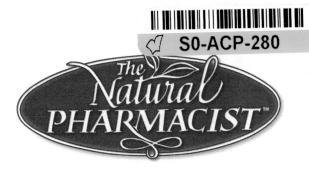

SO-ACP-280

The Natural PHARMACIST™

Everything You Need to Know About

Saw Palmetto and the Prostate

Anna M. Barton

Series Editors
Steven Bratman, M.D.
David Kroll, Ph.D.

Prima
HEALTH

A DIVISION OF PRIMA PUBLISHING
Visit us online at www.thenaturalpharmacist.com

Library of Congress Cataloging-in-Publication Data

Barton, Anna M.
  Saw palmetto and the prostate / Anna M. Barton.
    p.   cm.—(The natural pharmacist)
  Includes bibliographical references and index.
  ISBN 0-7615-1559-3
  1. Benign prostatic hyperplasia—treatment.   2. Saw palmetto—Therapeutic use.
  I. Title.   II. Series.
RC899.B37   1999
616.6'5—dc21
                                                                    98-49607
                                                                        CIP

00 01 02 HH 10 9 8 7 6 5 4 3
Printed in the United States of America

Visit us online at www.thenaturalpharmacist.com

Contents

What Makes This Book Different?   *vii*
Introduction   *xi*

1. What Is Saw Palmetto?   1

2. The Symptoms of Benign
   Prostatic Hyperplasia   11

3. What Causes Benign Prostatic Hyperplasia?   37

4. Conventional Surgical Treatment for BPH   49

5. Conventional Medical Treatment for BPH   69

6. Saw Palmetto: The Scientific Evidence   85

7. How to Take Saw Palmetto   105

8. Safety Issues   117

9. How Saw Palmetto Compares with
   Conventional Medications   125

10. Other Alternative Treatments for BPH   135

11. Putting It All Together   151

Notes   155
Index   169
About the Author and Series Editors   178

What Makes This Book Different?

The interest in natural medicine has never been greater. According to the National Association of Chain Drug Stores, 65 million Americans are using natural supplements, and the number is growing! Yet, it is hard for the consumer to find trustworthy sources for balanced information about this emerging field. Why? Frankly, natural medicine has had a checkered history. From snake oil potions sold at the turn of the century to those books, magazines, and product catalogs that hype miracle cures today, this is a field where exaggerated claims have been the norm. Proponents of natural medicine have tended to abuse science, treating it more as a marketing tool than a means of discovering the truth.

But there is truth to be found. Studies of vitamins, minerals, and other food supplements have been with us since these nutritional substances were first discovered, and the level and quality of this science has grown dramatically in the last 20 years. Herbal medicine has been neglected in the United States, but in Europe, this, the oldest of all healing arts, has been the subject of tremendous and ongoing scientific interest.

At present, for a number of herbs and supplements, it is possible to give reasonably scientific answers to the questions: How well does this work? How safe is it? What types of conditions is it best used for?

THE NATURAL PHARMACIST series is designed to cut through the hype and tell you what we know and what we don't know about popular natural treatments. These books are more conservative than any others available, more honest about the weaknesses of natural approaches, more fair in their comparisons of natural and conventional treatments. You won't find any miracle cures here, but you will discover useful options that can help you become healthier.

Why Choose Natural Treatments?

Although the science behind natural medicine continues to grow, this is still a much less scientifically validated field than conventional medicine. You might ask, "Why should I resort to an herb that is only partly proven, when I could take a drug with solid science behind it?" There are at least three good reasons to consider natural alternatives.

First, some herbs and supplements offer benefits that are not matched by any conventional drug. Vitamin E is a good example. It appears to help prevent prostate cancer, a benefit that no standard medication can claim. Also, vitamin E almost certainly helps prevent heart disease. While there are standard drugs that also prevent heart disease, vitamin E works differently and may be able to complement many of the other approaches.

Another example is the herb milk thistle. Studies strongly suggest that this herb can protect the liver from injury. There is no pill or tablet your doctor can prescribe to do the same.

Even if the science behind some of these treatments is less than perfect, when the risks are low and the possible benefit high, a natural treatment may be worth trying. It is a little-known fact that for many conventional treatments the science is less than perfect as well, and physicians must balance uncertain benefits against incompletely understood risks.

A second reason to consider natural therapies is that some may offer benefits comparable to those of drugs with fewer side effects. The herb St. John's wort is a good example. Reasonably strong scientific evidence suggests that this herb is an effective treatment for mild to moderate depression, while producing fewer side effects on average than conventional medications. Saw palmetto for benign enlargement of the prostate, ginkgo for relieving symptoms and perhaps slowing the progression of Alzheimer's disease, and glucosamine for osteoarthritis are other examples. This is not to say that herbs and supplements are completely harmless—they're not—but for most the level of risk is quite low.

Finally, there is a philosophical point to consider. For many people, it "feels" better to use a treatment that comes from nature instead of from a laboratory. Just as you might rather wear all-cotton clothing than polyester, or look at a mountain landscape rather than the skyscrapers of a downtown city, natural treatments may simply feel more compatible with your view of life. We can quibble endlessly about just what "natural" means and whether a certain treatment is "actually" natural or not, but such arguments are beside the point. The difference is in the feeling, and feelings matter. In fact, having a good feeling about taking an herb may lead you to use it more consistently than you would a prescription drug.

Of course, at times synthetic drugs may be necessary and even lifesaving. But on many other occasions it may be quite reasonable to turn to an herb or supplement instead of a drug.

To make good decisions you need good information. Unfortunately, while hundreds of books on alternative medicine are published every year, many are highly misleading.

The phrase "studies prove" is often used when the studies in question are so small or so badly conducted that they prove nothing at all. You may even find that the "data" from other books comes from studies with petri dishes and not real people!

You can't even assume that books written by well-known authors are scientifically sound. Many of these authors rely on secondary writers, leading to a game of "telephone," where misconceptions are passed around from book to book. And there's a strong tendency to exaggerate the power of natural remedies, whitewashing them with selective reporting.

THE NATURAL PHARMACIST series gives you the balanced information you need to make informed decisions about your health needs. Setting a new, high standard of accuracy and objectivity, these books take a realistic look at the herbs and supplements you read about in the news. You will encounter both favorable and unfavorable studies in these pages and will learn about both the benefits and the risks of natural treatments.

THE NATURAL PHARMACIST series is the source you can trust.

Steven Bratman, M.D.
David Kroll, Ph.D.

Introduction

Prostate enlargement, which affects the majority of men over the age of 50, can cause symptoms ranging from the mildly annoying to the seriously embarrassing. In rare cases, the side effects may even be life-threatening. If you have experienced the time-wasting inconvenience of frequent urination and diminished force of stream, the discomfort of feeling unable to empty your bladder, or have had your sleep disrupted by multiple nighttime trips to the bathroom, you could benefit from the information presented in this book.

The conventional treatment approaches for prostatic enlargement in the United States today include surgery and a few other procedures for removing or destroying the excess tissue. As well, there are now two types of pharmaceutical drugs approved by the FDA for treatment of this problem. While the drugs are often a better option than surgery, they are associated with a number of undesirable side effects. Dizziness, fainting, headaches, and loss of energy are some of the complaints known to occur with use of drugs such as Cardura and Hytrin, which are also used to treat hypertension. Flomax, a similar type of drug, causes a problem related to sexual function in around 18% of the people using it. Besides the fact that they have the potential to cause side effects, these drugs only treat the symptoms, not the cause. They do not decrease the size of the prostate.

The second type of drug available may get more to the heart of the problem. Proscar has received recent acclaim for its ability to actually shrink the prostate and possibly reduce the risk for needing surgery. However, like all drugs, it is also known to cause side effects. Impotence, loss of libido, ejaculatory dysfunction, growth of breast tissue, and rashes are seen in some of the men who use it. Even more worrisome, though, is that the use of Proscar may interfere with the method most often used to screen for prostate cancer—the prostate-specific antigen (PSA) level—which could potentially mask cancer from early detection.

While men in the United States are offered the alternatives of surgical procedures or drugs with these unpleasant side-effect profiles, men with prostate enlargement in Germany are usually placed on an herbal medicine by their physicians. The extract of saw palmetto berries has been found through clinical testing to be as effective in providing symptom relief as the pharmaceutical drugs available. The most serious side effect noted in trials, involving more than 2,000 participants over the last 30 years, is minor stomach upset. Furthermore, it appears to do what only one of the man-made drugs will do: shrink the prostate—without altering the results of tests used for cancer screening.

Oddly enough, the prescription most often used by doctors in Germany, and frequently in other countries throughout Europe as well, comes from a plant imported from the United States. Saw palmetto was used by American physicians for this purpose as recently as the 1940s, but was apparently forgotten as herbal medicines fell out of favor with the medical establishment.

Since then, however, laboratory and clinical tests have documented that saw palmetto extract, like the prescription drugs, can provide relief for around two-thirds of the men who try it. This book will fairly present the research that has been done on saw palmetto, provide information on conventional methods of treatment, and discuss what is known about the cause of the problem itself, allowing you to make better informed choices about your own health care. We believe the information will be both helpful and hopeful.

What Is Saw Palmetto?

If you shop regularly in health food stores, read magazines that cover the subject of herbal medicine, or see a naturopathic physician, you've probably already heard of the famous "prostate herb," saw palmetto. You may already know that this small fan palm tree that grows in the southeastern United States and the Caribbean is widely used in Europe as a treatment for benign prostatic hyperplasia, also called prostate enlargement or BPH for short. In this chapter, I will tell you more about this plant, what it looks like, what's in it, and how it has come to be so popular.

Saw palmetto has been described as having a height of as much as 20 feet in one text, an average height of 10 feet in another, and a height of 3 to 4 feet in yet another. Actually seeing the plant helps explain this lack of agreement. The species usually grows with its trunk along the ground for some distance before rising up to form foliage. Thus, it's entirely possible that the trunk could be 10 or even 20 feet in length, and the plant could still be 3 or 4 feet in

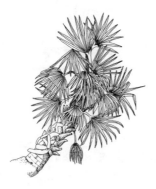

Figure 1. *Saw palmetto*

height. What you consider to be the height of the plant depends on how you perform your measurements.

The leaves are typical of a palm, with clusters of blade-like foliage branching out from a central point to form a fan, which is generally 2 feet or more in diameter (see figure 1).

The small tree produces white blossoms in clusters at the end of a stem that sprouts from the same point that the fans originate. The effect is similar to that of the blossoms of the common houseplant known as a spider plant. The flowers ripen into dark brown or black berries ranging from 1 to 2 centimeters in length.[1] It's this fruit that's used for treatment of BPH. We'll talk about the symptoms of this condition and how you can help it with saw palmetto and other natural treatments, such as nettle root, in later chapters.

Why Is It Called Saw Palmetto?

Saw palmetto is a plant called by many different names. It is known as saw palmetto because its leaves have serrate edges, like the teeth of a saw. Its Latin name is *Serenoa repens* but this plant is sometimes referred to as sabal, especially in Europe, which is taken from its other Latin name,

Sabal serrulata. It's also sometimes called American dwarf palm and scrub palm. In fact, there seems to be a lot of confusion about the plant's true name, both scientific and common. How, you might ask, can a plant have more than one scientific name?

It's fairly easy to understand how more than one common name could be given to the same plant by different groups of people. But aren't scientists supposed to be doing things more, well, scientifically? The fact that saw palmetto has more than one Latin name isn't really unique to this plant. When botanists assign a plant its Latin name, they first attempt to classify it correctly, using the categories many of us were asked to memorize back in our junior high biology classes: kingdom, phylum, class, order, family, genus, and species. Where the categories are broad (we knew it was a plant), the placement is fairly easy. However, by the time one has refined it down to the genus category, it gets trickier. An added complication is that when a new genus is discovered, it might be determined that the plant someone thought they had correctly labeled many years ago now seems to belong in a different category.

Saw palmetto has been used to treat a variety of complaints, from urinary tract infections to depressed libido.

Serenoa and *Sabal* are two genera belonging to the family *Palmae* (also known as *Arecaceae,* just in case it wasn't already confusing enough). *Sabal* was the genera in which the plant was first placed; however, because the palms in the genus *Sabal* are tall and tree-like, it was decided that the saw palmetto, a shorter, more scrub-like palm, belonged in *Serenoa.*[2]

How Did We Learn About Saw Palmetto?

The use of saw palmetto berries as a medicinal herb was probably learned by European settlers from Native Americans. Immigrants, arriving in a country lacking many of the herbs they were accustomed to using, had to adapt to their new environment, and they were greatly aided by the Native Americans, who had excellent knowledge of the medical use of the local plants. A settler named Nicolaes van Wassenaer, in a work published in 1624, wrote, "they have abundant means, with herbs and leaves or roots, to cure their ailments. There is not an ailment they have not a remedy for."

Regrettably, much of what was learned was never set to paper for one reason or another. In *History of North Carolina*, published in 1714, the author bemoans this, saying, "Amongst all the discoveries of America by the Missionaries of the French and Spaniards, I wonder none of them was so kind to the world

The second part of the scientific name, the species, describes the plant's characteristics. For example, *repens* means creeping, or prostrate, and refers to the way the trunk of the palm grows along the ground. The species name *serrulata* describes the serrate edges of the leaves.[3]

Of course, once the decision has been made to reclassify a plant, it takes some time for everyone to adjust. In fact, not everyone in the field of botany and the related scientific fields might agree. There's plenty of potential for even more confusion. In at least one text, the plant is referred to as *Serenoa serrulata*.

For clarity in this book, I'll use only the common name *saw palmetto* and the scientific name *Serenoa repens*.

as to have kept a catalogue of the distempers they found the savages capable of curing, and their method of cure, which might have been of some advantage to our *Materia Medica* at home."

This might have been partly due to the reluctance of the Native Americans to reveal the methods of healing that they used. In some tribes, the practice of medicine was directly tied into the practice of religion, and training in these skills was reserved for a few chosen members of the tribe. Dr. Johann David Schopf, a physician from Germany, came to America in the late 1700s and learned enough in his travels to write the *Materia Medica Americana.* In this book, he credits the Native Americans with great generosity and a willingness to provide "roots, barks, and herbs for the use of those needing aid, even if they do not indicate where they got them." You can almost sense his frustration, even 200 years after the fact.

However, should you choose to do more research on this plant's history and uses, be assured that other designations refer to the same plant.

What Is in Saw Palmetto?

For medicinal use, an extract of saw palmetto is made, composed primarily of fatty acids and sterols. If you really want the nitty-gritty details, a fatty acid is a carbon chain, usually with an even number of carbons, attached to a carboxyl (acidic) group on one end. The acidic end will associate with water while the rest of it will try to keep its distance. A sterol is a cyclic solid alcohol and one of the types of lipids

Recognition of Saw Palmetto

From the fragmentary history that's available on saw palmetto, we know that various parts of the plant were used by the Mayans for medicinal purposes, although no mention is made of the berries. Settlers in the American colonies in the late eighteenth century reported that both the Native Americans and the local wildlife used the berries as a food. The settlers attributed medicinal value to the fruit because of the apparent good health of the people and animals that consumed it.

It was not until 1906 that the plant was formally recognized as having therapeutic value and was listed in *The Pharmacopeia of the United States.* That listing was later moved to the *National Formulary,* which included saw palmetto until 1950. At this time, most of the herbal remedies were dropped from the *National*

commonly found in the membranes of plant cells. Cholesterol, which serves as the raw material that our bodies use to make many hormones, including testosterone, is also a sterol but is not found in plants. However, some of the sterols found in plants do have great chemical similarity to cholesterol and the various derivative hormones and are therefore biochemically active in our systems.[4] (For more information on cholesterol, see *The Natural Pharmacist Guide to Garlic and Cholesterol.*)

What Was Saw Palmetto Used for Historically?

Saw palmetto, being indigenous to the North American continent, was valued for its healing properties by the Native American population. Many uses for the plant are found

Formulary, probably because of the medical community's growing preference for pharmaceutical drugs.[5] However, it was going to be quite a while before any drugs would come along that worked as well as saw palmetto for BPH. *The Dispensatory of the United States of America* also came to include information on saw palmetto, noting it to be useful in the treatment of chronic and subacute cystitis (bladder infection) and "especially recommended in cases of enlarged prostate."[6] The author of the *Dispensatory* states his belief that it's unlikely that the herb directly affected the prostate, believing it to relieve symptoms only, which he attributed to relaxation of the mucous membranes lining the urethra. As we shall see, he wasn't entirely right. Saw palmetto does appear to affect the prostate directly.

in historical literature, with virtually all its parts being used—the leaves, roots, and bark as well as the berries. It has been used for ailments such as dysentery and stomach pains, both of which are treated with a tea made from the leaves and roots. It has also been used as poultices, made from the bark of the tree, for wounds and bites. The berries are noted to have been used to treat a wide variety of genital and urinary complaints, ranging from urinary tract infections to depressed libido. As well, the fruit is credited as a sedative, an aid to digestion, an expectorant, and a treatment for infertility, painful menstruation, and an agent in increasing milk production and breast size in women.[7]

Whenever I see a plant that claims to have that many uses, I'm a bit skeptical. It's too reminiscent of patent medicines that once were sold from the back of a wagon. How can you know which claims are valid?

Luckily for men with benign prostatic hyperplasia (BPH), saw palmetto has been studied as a therapy for this condition for many years, both in laboratory experiments and in clinical trials. Not only is there plenty of evidence to show that it does work as a treatment for BPH, but there are studies investigating the biochemical mechanisms by which this is accomplished. I'll discuss the studies that have been done and the current thinking about the mechanism (or mechanisms) of action in chapter 6.

Current Uses of Saw Palmetto

Saw palmetto is widely used today for treatment of BPH in European countries including Italy, France, Spain, and Germany, as well as in New Zealand. In Germany, herbal remedies are used more often for this condition than pharmaceutical drugs, and saw palmetto is one of the main herbal options (along with nettle and beta-sitosterol). Indeed, herbs are a standard against which new treatments are evaluated. When a new drug for BPH comes out, researchers in Europe are likely to compare it against saw palmetto extract to see if it is worth putting on the market.

Saw palmetto has been studied for many years, both in laboratory experiments and in clinical trials.

Before using any treatment for BPH, whether herbal or pharmaceutical, you need to be absolutely certain that you have the disease correctly identified by a physician. In the following chapter, I'll provide detailed information on the symptoms, their causes, and the methods used to obtain an accurate diagnosis.

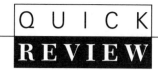

- Saw palmetto, a small fan palm native to southeastern Atlantic and Gulf coast areas of the United States, produces berries that possess medicinal properties useful in the treatment of prostate enlargement.

- Although saw palmetto is called by such names as *Sabal serrulata*, sabal, and different variations of palm, its currently accepted scientific name is *Serenoa repens* (the name used to refer to it throughout this book).

- For medicinal use, an extract is made of saw palmetto that contains many fatty acids and lesser amounts of plant sterols (substances similar to cholesterol).

- Saw palmetto extract is one of the standard treatments for benign prostatic hyperplasia (BPH) in Europe, and new drugs are often compared against existing herbal medications to see if they are worth putting on the market.

- Before using any form of treatment for symptoms of BPH, you need to have an accurate diagnosis of your condition.

The Symptoms
of Benign Prostatic
Hyperplasia

I f you are male, odds are your life will someday be complicated by prostate problems. If you are female, the chances are very high that someone you know and care about will eventually be affected by these disorders. In this chapter, we'll explore the symptoms you, or someone you know, might experience with benign prostatic hyperplasia (BPH). If you'd prefer to read about natural treatments for BPH right away, turn to chapters 6, 7, and 10 in which we'll discuss the evidence for saw palmetto and other herbal and nutritional approaches.

By the age of 60, 50% of men will develop benign prostatic hyperplasia, a noncancerous but excessive growth of the prostate. Beyond the age of 80, 90% of the male population have prostate enlargement. However, only about half the men who have this condition will experience symptoms. As we will see in later chapters, saw palmetto appears to provide effective relief for many of these symptoms.

Andrew's Story

Andrew hadn't slept through the night for many months. Neither had his wife, Barbara. Three or four times a night, sometimes more, he had to get up to relieve himself. Finally, there came a night when Barbara asked him to sleep on the sofa.

She was contrite at breakfast.

"Andrew," she said, "I wish you'd go see the doctor about this."

"Barbara, I'm sure it's no big deal."

"Well, I think it could be. Elsa told me her husband David was having the same problems. He went in to see their doctor about it, and they told him he had enlargement of the prostate."

Andrew started to open his mouth to speak, but Barbara continued.

"He was doing just the same things you've been doing, Andrew. Getting up five or six times a night, having to go every hour or so during the day. Going and then having to go again

What Is the Prostate?

Unlike the major organs, the prostate's function, and even its location, might not be familiar to everyone. Before proceeding to a discussion of the symptoms and treatment of BPH, let's take a look at the structure and function of the prostate.

The prostate is a gland that lies tucked up against the lower surface of the bladder. Although it has been described as being similar in size to a golf ball or a walnut, I would liken it to a strawberry, as this gives a somewhat more accurate image of its shape. The prostate surrounds five minutes later. So they put him on some kind of medication, and he's doing a lot better, Elsa says."

He thought about it a moment.

"If you didn't have to be up and down all night, don't you think you'd feel better?" Barbara asked.

"Well, I suppose," Andrew answered.

Barbara wasted no time in getting him an appointment, which turned out to be a good thing. It was just what she had thought—his prostate was enlarged. Benign prostatic hyperplasia, they called it. Turned out, the doctor told him, that this happens to most men as they get older—more than half over 50, and almost everyone over 80.

The medications the doctor prescribed took a few weeks to start working, but Andrew was starting to notice a little improvement, and that was enough to let both him and Barbara sleep a little easier.

the urethra—the tube that conducts urine from the bladder out to the tip of the penis. It also encompasses the ejaculatory ducts as they join with the urethra.

In addition to acting as the conduit for urine, the urethra is the route used by seminal fluids, which are made up of sperm from the testes and of secretions produced by the seminal vesicles and the prostate gland. Prostate secretions can account for as much as one-third of the total volume of ejaculate produced during orgasm. This alkaline fluid plays a role in sperm activation.[1]

The prostate is conically shaped (see figure 2), broader at the end closest to the bladder, and narrows slightly at the

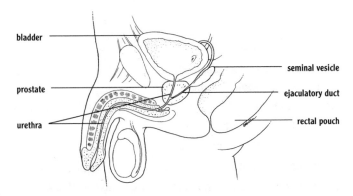

Figure 2. *Cross section showing the prostate and its relationship to other organs*

end nearer the base of the penis. Although it might seem backwards, the top (broader) end of the prostate is referred to in medical terminology as the *base* and the lower end as the *apex*. At this narrower end, the prostate joins with the urethral sphincter, the muscle that you use to voluntarily control the flow of urine. At the base, the muscles that form the neck of the bladder act to prevent semen from *refluxing*, or traveling in the wrong direction, up into the bladder during an ejaculation. The muscles of the prostate itself contract during an orgasm and help to propel the seminal fluids outward through the urethra.

Divisions of the Prostate

Three lobes make up the prostate: the left and right lateral lobes, with the urethra dividing them, and the smaller, middle lobe, which is the portion above the intersection of the ejaculatory ducts and the urethra and lying behind the urethra.

The prostate is also described as having different "zones" based on the composition and developmental origin of the glandular tissues within it (see figure 3). At the center, in a position within the prostate similar to that of a pit within an avocado, and surrounding the urethra is the transition zone. In a normal prostate, this tissue makes up only 5 to 10% of the total tissue. It is in this zone that BPH most often occurs. As well, around 20% of all prostate cancers originate here.

The central zone of the prostate is a roughly cone-shaped portion of tissue. Its narrower tip meets the urethra next to the apex end of the transition zone, which surrounds the ejaculatory ducts at the point where they join with the urethra. It borders the underside of the transition zone, then extends along the underside of the urethra up to the base of the prostate. It surrounds the ejaculatory ducts from their point of entry into the prostate to their junction with the urethra.

Outside both of the other zones and forming the bulk of a normal, healthy prostate is the peripheral zone. It accounts for 70% of the tissue of a normal prostate and is also where 70% of prostate cancers begin. Part of the peripheral zone can be felt by your doctor during a rectal exam, as described later in this chapter.

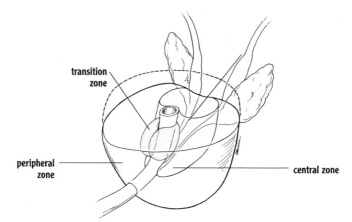

Figure 3. *Prostate zones*

Tissues That Make Up the Prostate

The prostate is made up of about 70% glandular tissue and 30% smooth muscle and connective tissues. The muscular and connective tissues provide structural support for the secretory cells and allow the prostate to contract. A thin, membranous layer called the *capsule* surrounds all the other prostate tissues.[2]

What Is Prostatic Fluid?

The prostate produces about 30% of the volume of fluid emitted during ejaculation. One purpose of the secretions is to lubricate and cleanse the urethra prior to the passage of the semen. Prostatic fluid has a very high zinc content, and research suggests that this serves as an antibacterial agent to help prevent infections. As well, the prostatic fluid is much more alkaline than the sperm or the seminal secretions, raising the pH of semen to about 7.5. This increase in alkalinity increases the motility of the sperm and might protect it in the more acidic environment of the vagina during fertilization.

The Seminal Vesicles

The seminal vesicles lie above the prostate in back of the bladder. The *vas deferens,* which carry sperm from the testes, join the ducts from the seminal vesicles just before entering the prostate, where the combined tubes become known as the *ejaculatory ducts.* The intersection that allows the urethra to be used for both elimination and reproduction occurs at the end of the transition zone toward the base of the penis.

Normal Growth and Development

During boyhood, the prostate, like most other structures involved in male reproduction, is much smaller than in adulthood. The production of the hormone testosterone in the testes increases dramatically with the onset of adolescence. This hormone is released into the bloodstream, where it circulates throughout the body.

Those tissues that have *androgen receptors* respond to testosterone directly or by converting it to another form first. Androgens are hormones that have a masculinizing effect. The receptors for these can be described as hormone-specific docking areas that exist within the cell. Only a molecule with the right structure fits, or *binds,* into this site.

The prostate converts testosterone into another androgen, dihydrotestosterone (DHT). It does this by manufacturing an enzyme, 5-alpha-reductase, which causes a chemical reaction that alters the testosterone. The DHT binds to receptor sites within the prostatic cells, triggering cell division and resulting in growth of the prostate. The prostate will nearly double in size by adulthood. DHT and the enzyme 5-alpha-reductase also

By the age of 60, 50% of men will develop benign prostatic hyperplasia, a noncancerous but excessive growth of the prostate.

appear to play a part in the growth that results in BPH. Blocking this conversion of testosterone into DHT has been the focus of one of the pharmaceutical drugs (finasteride, also known as Proscar) currently being used for treatment.

There is evidence that saw palmetto might also affect this pathway.[3–7] We'll talk more about how saw palmetto might help BPH in chapter 6.

A Natural Part of Aging?

There is some disagreement as to whether BPH should be considered a disease. Because BPH is so common, it almost seems to be a natural part of aging and is perhaps becoming more problematic because we are living longer. Yet the growth due to BPH differs from normal developmental growth in that it produces small lumps, or *nodules*, that are usually concentrated within the transition zone, as mentioned earlier. Is it a tumor or just a large prostate? There's no consensus just how to describe it.[8]

Prostate growth due to BPH differs from normal developmental growth in that it produces small lumps.

Not too surprisingly, given the lack of agreement regarding what BPH really is, the cause or causes of BPH are still somewhat mysterious to modern medical science. Several theories exist, and research investigating these is ongoing. I'll go into more detail about what's known and what's being explored in the next chapter. First, let's discuss the symptoms of BPH.

Signs and Symptoms of BPH

The following problems can be symptoms of BPH, although other causes are possible. I'll describe the meanings of the terms most often used by doctors for these complaints, as well as why BPH could cause these to happen. As we shall see in chapter 6, good evidence suggests that saw palmetto may relieve most of these symptoms. Other herbs that might also be effective include pygeum, nettle root, grass pollen extract, and beta-sitosterols from *Hypoxis rooperi* (see chapter 10).

Decreased Force and Stream of Urine

As the prostate grows, the additional tissue places pressure on the urethra. Additionally, the muscular portion of the prostate tenses up, perhaps in response to overcrowding or to biochemical signals. Both of these factors cause the opening through which your urine must pass to narrow, resulting in a slower, weaker stream, which means it may take you longer to *void,* or empty, your bladder. As we shall see in chapter 6, saw palmetto appears to reduce prostate size and may also relax muscles in the prostate. This would reduce the pressure on the urethra and may explain saw palmetto's documented benefits in BPH.

Postvoid Dribbling

Tissue blocking the urethra can prevent the urine remaining in the urethra from being returned to the bladder, as it normally is. Instead, the urine leaks out. This can be an annoying symptom, even if your BPH symptoms never become so severe that they warrant treatment. *Campbell's Urology* suggests compressing the penis along the shaft with your fingers to "milk" the residual urine out and blotting with toilet tissue.[9]

Hesitancy

The normal period between the time you voluntarily relax the urethral sphincter muscles to allow urine to pass and the time that your stream begins is usually a matter of seconds. If you find that you're waiting longer than you've had to in the past, this could also be an early symptom of BPH.

Interrupted Stream/Intermittency

A urine flow that haphazardly stops and restarts is also a common early symptom of an obstructed urethra. Such an obstruction can be caused by BPH, and the stop-and-go urination is typically due to intermittent blocking of the urethra by prostate growth.

Urinary Retention

The bladder is not just a sack that holds urine until you permit it to pass; rather, it's composed of muscular tissue that compresses to expel the urine. Ideally, this should allow you to completely empty your bladder. One of your body's first responses to the narrowing of the urethra is to increase the amount of force your bladder applies. This is one of the reasons that BPH (or cancer) can go undetected until it's fairly progressed.

If you don't have BPH, you might need to urinate once or twice during the night; however, greater frequency is a classic BPH symptom.

Exercising the muscle used to express urine, the detrusor muscle, eventually causes it to increase in size and decrease in flexibility. When too much of the urethra is blocked, the bladder might be unable to apply enough force to empty completely, leaving residual urine within it. This can leave you with a (valid) sensation of incomplete emptying and also lead to further complications (see Acute Urinary Retention).

Some researchers suggest that saw palmetto may work like alpha-blocker drugs and relax the opening of the bladder, which might increase the volume of urine released and allow the bladder to empty more completely. We'll discuss this more in-depth in chapter 6.

Straining

If you find yourself trying to compress the bladder using your abdominal muscles at any time other than the very end of urination, it might be an indication that you have some urethral obstruction. Without such obstruction, the bladder itself should be capable of applying adequate pressure.

Increased Urinary Frequency

When the bladder fails to empty completely, there's less volume to fill before you again feel the need to urinate, causing you to make more frequent trips to the bathroom. Also, with the thickening and strengthening of the muscle tissue in the bladder that occurs over time, called *trabeculation,* the bladder becomes less pliable and less able to stretch to accommodate greater volumes. Its capacity to hold urine is reduced, and, as it remains partially filled, you end up needing to relieve yourself far more often.

Nocturia

If you don't have BPH, you might need to void once or twice during the night, especially if you've consumed a lot of liquid before bedtime. However, greater frequency is a classic symptom of the illness. *Nocturia* (a fancy name for this nighttime call of nature) could also result from some other, seemingly unrelated conditions (such as heart and circulatory problems). A visit to see your doctor is in order if you find yourself making that journey down the hall more than two or three times a night on a regular basis.

Dysuria

Pain felt while urinating, or *dysuria,* can result either from the physical pressure caused by the blockage or from inflammation associated with bladder infections. Infections can occur more frequently with BPH because the urine remains in the bladder longer, providing more opportunity for organisms to grow. It's also possible that because your urine stream is diminished, you're not washing out the urethra as effectively, allowing bacteria to invade. *Strangury,* pain at the end of urination, is another symptom usually related to bladder infections.

Hematuria

Blood in the urine, or *hematuria,* can accompany BPH. It could also be a possible symptom of an infection caused by BPH. As with most of these symptoms, there are other possible causes as well. For example, hematuria could be a sign of bladder cancer. In order to nourish the cells produced by cancer, your body may start forming excessive amounts of blood vessels (known as increased vascularization). A bladder infection can also cause bleeding. This is a symptom that demands immediate medical attention to see if it is due to BPH or something else.

Urgency

Along with causing blockage of the urethra, BPH has the potential to affect the muscles that control the flow of urine. Some BPH sufferers experience the sudden need to be in the bathroom instantly. Failure to make it there before leakage occurs is referred to as *urge incontinence,* a potentially embarrassing symptom. *Enuresis,* or bed-wetting, is a similarly disturbing effect of the loss of muscular control.

Other possible causes for urgency include bladder infections, nervous system disorders, and anxiety (which itself can be an indirect symptom of BPH).

Acute Urinary Retention

I placed this symptom in its own category, rather than including it with more moderate symptoms of urinary retention, because it's the only symptom of BPH that's immediately life-threatening. With acute urinary retention it isn't just hard to urinate, it's nearly impossible. This symptom can occur progressively, following symptoms of blockage that worsen over time, or it can have a sudden and unexpected onset. There have been cases of men with BPH who were entirely without symptoms until suddenly one day they had a complete restriction of the flow of urine, but this is rare. Ingestion of large amounts of alcohol or the use of antihistamines like Benadryl (diphenhydramine) as well as other anticholinergics, Sudafed (pseudoephedrine) or other sympathomimetic decongestants like phenylpropanolamine, and general anesthesia have been known to accelerate a sudden onset of symptoms.

The only symptom of BPH that's immediately life-threatening is acute urinary retention, the complete or nearly complete inability to urinate.

Whether occurring suddenly or over a period of time, acute urinary retention constitutes a medical emergency and requires immediate treatment. The pressure of the

Is It BPH or Prostate Cancer?
See Your Doctor to Be Sure!

Whether your prostate problems are first detected in a routine examination or noticed by you in the form of symptoms, you should find out as much as possible about the source of the trouble as soon as possible. Because both BPH and prostate cancer result in an overgrowth of prostate tissue, the symptoms can be quite similar. For this reason, it's extremely important that you should see your doctor to discover which you have. BPH is mostly an annoyance, although perhaps a great one, but prostate cancer can kill you. However, with early detection of prostate cancer before it has had a chance to spread, the chances of a

urine, unable to pass at all, can rupture the bladder or back up into the kidneys, causing kidney failure and possibly death. However, this complication is fairly easily treated if you see your doctor right away.

Absence of Symptoms

I mentioned earlier that BPH does not cause symptoms in all men who have it. Surprisingly, there's no apparent correlation between the size of a man's prostate and the development of symptoms. You'd think that the bigger the prostate the worse the symptoms. However, this isn't true. You could have a significantly enlarged prostate but experience only few or no symptoms, or you might have little enlargement and suffer from more severe problems. The complete cure are excellent. The 5-year survival rate for men with prostate cancer that's still confined to the prostate is 100%. That's a very encouraging number! However, the rub is "early detection." The same set of statistics from the American Cancer Society indicates an 89% 5-year survival rate for all men found to have prostate cancer, meaning that 11% were not detected early and led to death.[10] You do not want to be in that 11%! Seeing a doctor at the first sign of BPH symptoms could save your life. (For more information on cancer, see *The Natural Pharmacist Guide to Reducing Cancer Risk*.)

real issue is whether the enlarged prostate is squeezing the urethra or not. Sometimes, there's a lot of "wiggle room" and even significant prostatic hyperplasia might not cause any symptoms. Thus, you could have BPH for years, and it might not ever bother you. If this is the case, "watchful waiting" is usually recommended, meaning that no treatment is prescribed, but regular checkups are done to monitor the progress of the condition.

It's quite unusual, with our society's growing awareness of the prevalence of prostate problems and the need for routine examinations, for BPH to go undetected. Deaths from complications of BPH in the United States are extremely rare. They generally occur only in people who can't afford health maintenance care or who actually choose to avoid medical treatment.

An Overview of Methods
Used to Diagnose BPH

Alone, none of the tests used to diagnose prostate problems can give absolute answers. Therefore, your doctor will probably use some combination of the following methods. You might think of it in terms of observing a sculpture—you need to see it from several different angles before you can really describe it.

Measurements of your urine's flow rate and the amount of urine being retained in the bladder will help determine the degree of obstruction and help track your progress, with or without treatment. Observing what is in the urine, using both chemical tests and examination under a microscope, will help determine whether you have an infection and, if so, where the infection is located. If the blockage has been severe enough to cause damage to the kidneys, this can also begin to reveal itself through urinalysis.

Suprisingly, there's no apparent correlation between the size of a man's prostate and the development of BPH symptoms.

Physical examination and hearing the subjective symptoms of the patient—what he has personally felt and observed—are very important parts of the groundwork for making a diagnosis. Your doctor might give you a formal questionnaire to complete that will help assess symptom severity and provide a baseline for progress checks.

Blood samples can be analyzed for certain proteins that will yield information about your prostate's size and condition and your kidneys' functioning. Blood work can also be useful in identifying an infection.

Imaging studies, which allow us to see the inner workings of the body without surgery, are often done along with the other tests to get a more precise idea of the size and location of any growth of the prostate. Some of these methods help determine whether a cancer has spread, and others are used to measure the quantity of retained urine present.

Finally, if cancer is suspected, biopsies of tissue samples are used to make a final determination.

Urodynamics

Knowing the velocity, volume, and pressure of your urine stream helps gauge the degree of obstruction. A specialized device called a uroflow meter can measure these. Although this information doesn't necessarily aid in determining why the blockage is present (e.g., whether it's caused by BPH, prostate cancer, or some foreign body), it can be very useful in measuring the success of a treatment protocol.

Urinalysis

Your urine yields a surprising amount of information about your health. The "dipstick" typically used in your doctor's office—that little piece of paper with the different colored squares—can monitor for glucose, bilirubin, ketones, specific gravity, blood, protein, bacteria, pH, urobilinogen, leukocytes, and nitrites. Most of these screen for diseases not related to the prostate, but the presence of blood or bacteria can indicate a bladder infection, which can, as mentioned, be a symptom related to blockage.

Digital Rectal Exam

If you are male and 50 years or older, it's recommended that a digital rectal exam (DRE) be a part of your regular physical exam. Your doctor will insert a rubber-gloved and lubricated finger into the anal canal to feel the area of the prostate that comes into contact with the rectal wall. Only part of the prostate can be felt directly this way, but it's in this portion that 70% of all prostate cancers begin. This exam, although not definitive, is considered a valuable diagnostic tool.

Because the symptoms of BPH and prostate cancer can be similar, it's important you see your doctor to discover which you have.

A normal prostate will feel smooth and slightly elastic to the touch. Subtle changes in texture, shape, and symmetry can be detected by a health professional who's familiar with this exam. A prostate that is infected or inflamed can have a softer, squishier texture, often described as *boggy.* An enlarged prostate might be noticed as being enlarged during the exam or might just feel firmer than usual. If you've developed cancer in the portion of the prostate nearest to the anal cavity, your doctor might notice lumpiness, or *nodularity,* of the tissue. However, it's possible for BPH or cancer to go undetected by a DRE.

During the exam, the slight pressure placed on the prostate can cause some of the prostatic fluid to be squeezed out of the prostate and pass through the urethral duct. This fluid sample can be examined for bacteria or blood to aid in diagnosing bacterial prostatitis (prostate infection). If a urine sample is taken both before and after the exam, this too can help determine the site of an infection. The presence of bacteria in the urine prior to the exam likely indicates that the infection is in the bladder or possibly the kidneys. If, on the other hand, the first specimen is clear but the second reveals bacterial contamination, the prostate itself is probably infected; the prostatic fluid released during the examination spreads the bacteria through the urethra so that it is revealed in the urine. Saw palmetto has occasionally been used to treat prostatitis, but pygeum, another herb used to treat BPH, is more often prescribed. However, there is little scientific evidence that either one is effective for prostate infection.

Prostate-Specific Antigen Testing

Your prostate manufactures a protein known as *prostate-specific antigen* (PSA). A bit of this protein normally escapes into the bloodstream and can be detected in a blood sample. With a healthy prostate, PSA levels usually increase in proportion with the size of the prostate. Because most men experience BPH as they age, it's generally considered normal for an older man to have a slightly higher PSA level than a younger man. However, if you have prostate cancer that has advanced far enough, the amount of PSA that leaks into your bloodstream increases beyond what would normally be expected with BPH.

A more accurate interpretation of PSA can be made by taking other factors into account. Some urologists use a combination of PSA and transrectal ultrasound (discussed later) to obtain a number referred to as the *PSA density*. This is the ratio of the mass of your prostate and the amount of PSA in your bloodstream. If the PSA level is abnormally high relative to prostate size, cancer might be present.

Another thing that doctors watch for is a sudden elevation in PSA levels. Extremely high PSAs, especially if greatly increased since your last PSA sample was drawn, could indicate that a cancer has already begun to spread to other places in the body. The comparison of your PSA from a previous exam with the current level is called *PSA velocity*.

The PSA in your blood can be found either floating around all by itself—*free PSA*—or joined together with another protein—*bound,* or *complexed, PSA.* A noncancerous individual will tend to have more free PSA relative to the total amount of PSA found in the bloodstream than someone who has prostate cancer. There are, however, some conflicting reports about the accuracy of this method of interpretation.

Your PSA can be affected by the medications prescribed for BPH. Proscar was shown in a 1996 study to decrease the PSA readings far more than it decreased the size of the prostate.[11] In the same study, standardized saw palmetto extract had no effect on PSA. There has been some concern that by artificially lowering PSA, Proscar might mask prostate cancer. It's comforting to see that this isn't one of the effects of saw palmetto, and is an argument for using it instead of Proscar. Otherwise, the two treatments were found to be equally effective in relieving the symptoms of BPH in the 1,098 men involved in the study. Proscar does have some advantages of its own, however. You can find more details on this in chapter 6.

Creatinine Measurement

Creatinine is a protein normally found in the bloodstream; however, higher-than-normal levels usually indicate that your kidneys aren't doing their job as well as they should. Measurement of creatinine is useful in determining whether a man with symptoms of *prostatism* (obstruction of the neck of the bladder due to an enlarged prostate) has begun to suffer *renal insufficiency*—kidney damage—as a result of the obstruction.

Transrectal Ultrasound

A transrectal ultrasound allows your doctor to see an image of your prostate. An ultrasound image is created when high-frequency sound waves are reflected back in the direction of the source as echoes. The returning vibrations are interpreted as an image by computer on the basis of the time it takes for them to return to the point of origin. The image is then displayed on a video screen.

Transrectal ultrasound (TRUS) uses a wand-shaped *transducer* to send and receive the ultrasound emissions to the prostate through the rectal wall. An anesthetic lubricant can be used during placement of the wand to minimize discomfort. The size and shape of the prostate can be determined, and in some cases the type of growth (cancerous or noncancerous) is identifiable. Denser tissue, in which cells are packed closer together, shows up on an ultrasound as a dark spot, referred to as *hypoechoic.* This characteristic is typical of cancerous tissue and produces the hard nodules that your doctor observes when performing a DRE. However, some cancers might take a different form and can avoid detection. Furthermore, there is a high frequency of false alarms with this test.

Still, TRUS is very useful in detecting nodules that can't be felt during an exam, and it can help rule out cancer in the case of BPH. The technology is also used in performing needle biopsies, which are often done simultaneously with this type of ultrasound imaging.

Transabdominal Ultrasound

Using the same technology as TRUS, an ultrasound image taken through the abdomen allows the doctor to see the prostate from a different angle. It can also be used to see how much residual urine is in the bladder following voiding and to observe changes in your bladder wall, kidneys, and upper urinary tract that can result from prolonged blockage.

Cystoscopy

A sophisticated piece of equipment, the cystoscope allows a urologist to see directly inside you by passing this tool through the urethra. With this device, the channel's inner walls and precise areas of blockage, the inside of the bladder, and the prostate can be viewed, allowing the urologist to estimate prostate size. The procedure can be useful in determining the cause of blood in the urine and for visualizing lesions or stones. It is also used prior to prostate surgery.

Intravenous Pyelogram

Used in conjunction with x ray, an intravenous pyelogram (IVP) involves receiving an injection of a "dye" that usually contains iodine. The dye is filtered by the kidneys and excreted. X rays taken while the dye is being processed for elimination show the kidneys, ureters (the tubes leading from the kidneys to the bladder), the bladder, and the urethra. It has been routinely used in men with prostate problems to determine the amount of urine being retained and to what degree the urethra is blocked. It can also show the structural changes in the bladder that result when increased pressure is needed to expel urine through the narrowing urethra.

Acute renal failure is known to occur in a very small percentage of people (less than 0.5%) following this procedure. The exact reasons for this are not known, but those at higher risk include those with a history of kidney failure, people with diabetes, the elderly, patients with dehydration, and those with multiple myelomas (a form of cancer).[12] Because the dyes used for IVP usually contain iodine, if you have a sensitivity to iodine, you should discuss this with your doctor if an IVP is suggested. Obviously, it's a tool that should be used only when absolutely necessary.

A similar procedure, called a *cystogram,* works on the same principles, but the dye is injected directly into the bladder through a catheter. This doesn't give an x-ray image of the kidneys or ureters unless there's a problem with reflux, in which the urine is being pushed backward up the ducts. However, not having the dye pass through the kidneys makes this procedure safer.

Computerized Tomography

Computerized tomography (CT) takes x-ray images in "slices" through a series of planes of your body and sends these images to a computer that assembles them to produce a three-dimensional image. The process is generally more expensive than an ultrasound or IVP, but in some cases it can yield information not as clearly produced by the other two.

Magnetic Resonance Imaging

Magnetic resonance imaging (MRI) also produces a three-dimensional image and is especially good for viewing soft tissue. However, it's also quite expensive and requires that you spend time in a small, enclosed space. There are possible hazards for individuals with implanted metal. For example, if you have a pacemaker, surgical pins, or imbedded shrapnel, you should discuss this with your doctor if an MRI is suggested.

Biopsy

If two or more of the tests above have given your doctor cause to suspect prostate cancer, a biopsy might be required to make a final determination. A tissue sample is taken from the prostate and then sent to the pathology laboratory for evaluation of the cell types found in it. This can be done while performing ultrasound, allowing your doctor to see precisely from which area the sample is being obtained. If ultrasound has revealed dense nodules that the doctor suspects are cancerous growths, this tissue will be wanted for biopsy.

Taking an Active Role in Your Treatment

The differences in opinion among general practice physicians, urologists, and even medical and public health organizations as to which diagnostic procedures and treatments to use for prostate problems are extreme. Whereas one doctor might state that cystoscopy is a standard and very useful technique, another might say that it's not helpful at all. There are similar discrepancies regarding the use of MRI, CT, IVP, and probably most of the methods just described. A study published in November 1997 in the *British Journal of Urology* showed the diagnosis of BPH to be one of the two problem areas with the least degree of consensus among urological experts and that diagnostic costs could vary by as much as 400%.[13]

To add to the confusion, I've found that many texts on prostate disease, even those written by doctors, will often state opinions as facts. My recommendation, if you want to educate yourself regarding your options, is to visit a medical library. Some hospitals maintain libraries that are available to the public. Medical reference texts and journals are more rigorously reviewed for accuracy than books written for laypersons, and, although perhaps less entertaining, they might give you more solid information.

If you have any questions about the procedures that your doctor is recommending, discuss it with him or her. Keep reading and asking questions until you're satisfied with your understanding. If your doctor is unwilling to spend this time answering your questions or is insisting on diagnostic methods that you disagree with, a second opinion might be in order. As well, many insurance carriers require a second opinion before some of the more expensive diagnostic techniques are used.

If your doctor determines that your condition is BPH and, after reading this book, you feel that saw palmetto might be the right alternative for you, I strongly encourage talking about this with him or her as well. Bring this book along, if you like, to show your doctor that there's scientific evidence supporting saw palmetto's use as a treatment for BPH. This might be a good starting place for a discussion, especially if he or she is unfamiliar with saw palmetto and its benefits.

An Expert Diagnosis Is Critical

The information in this book is intended to provide you with information that will broaden the range of choices that you can make with regard to treatment of BPH. However, it can't replace the care of a physician. An evaluation by a licensed medical practitioner, someone who is able to perform diagnostic testing such as that described here, is *absolutely necessary* to determine whether the symptoms you're experiencing are from BPH or from cancer of the prostate.

Cancer of the prostate *cannot* be treated with saw palmetto. If you're experiencing any of the symptoms described in this chapter, *do not* self-treat with saw palmetto without seeing your doctor. Relief of your symptoms with saw palmetto, or with any of the other herb treatments, would not be positive evidence that your symptoms were caused by BPH.

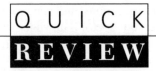

- Benign prostatic hyperplasia (BPH) is a noncancerous, but excessive, growth of the prostate gland.
- Although not life-threatening, BPH can become very uncomfortable, and the symptoms it can cause can be serious if not treated.
- BPH affects 50% of men between the ages of 51 and 60 and 90% of those 80 and older.
- The signs and symptoms of BPH include decreased force and stream of urine, postvoid dribbling, hesitancy, interrupted stream/ intermittency, urinary retention, straining, increased urinary frequency, nocturia, dysuria, hematuria, urgency, and acute urinary retention.
- *Note:* A diagnosis from a medical professional is absolutely necessary before treating your condition because prostate cancer and BPH have identical symptoms, and cancer can't be treated with saw palmetto.

What Causes Benign Prostatic Hyperplasia?

T he cause of BPH remains at least in part undiscovered. Actually, there are probably many causes at work. We have several pieces of the puzzle but as yet no complete picture.

Aging is the most easily identified factor involved in the development of BPH, because the number of men who have the problem increases dramatically with age, and it occurs almost exclusively in men after the age of 40. However, since we can't stop aging (yet), this observation is not terribly useful when it comes to inventing new treatments for BPH.

A more useful clue that medical practitioners have identified is that men can only develop BPH if they have working testes.[1] Based on this observation, the drastic act of surgical castration was briefly tried for the treatment of prostatic overgrowth in the late nineteenth and early twentieth centuries. Although it seemed to work, castration is obviously too extreme except to be used as a last resort for a life-threatening condition. Because BPH is now quite treatable, castration for this problem is, thankfully, a relic of past medical practice.

However, since not every man with functional testes develops BPH as he ages, there's more at work here. As you read through the following theories that are being investigated, I think you'll notice that many seem to connect with the others, like interlocking parts of a jigsaw puzzle. As I said earlier, the puzzle isn't solved yet, but researchers have found some of the right pieces.

Dihydrotestosterone and Prostate Growth

One of the many pieces of the prostate puzzle involves the role dihydrotestosterone plays in development of BPH. As you

The number of men who have BPH increases dramatically with age, and it occurs almost exclusively in men after the age of 40.

might recall from chapter 2, the prostate responds to a slightly altered version of the hormone testosterone, dihydrotestosterone (DHT), which binds to receptor sites within the prostate cells. It's known to be involved with the growth and development of the prostate during development and puberty.

It was suspected for a time that increased amounts of DHT in the prostate were the cause of BPH. Some research seemed to show that men with BPH had a higher concentration of DHT in the prostatic tissue than men without this condition. It has since been found that this is not the case. Even so, it's obvious that DHT does play a part in the occurrence of BPH.

Who Says It's Benign?

Benign might very well seem like a misnomer to anyone suffering from the symptoms of this all-too-common and highly unpleasant condition. Although in ordinary use the word usually refers to something harmless, in medical use it means a type of growth that is not cancerous. Still, the overgrowth of tissue can cause great discomfort and other complications that can become serious if left unchecked.

The term *benign prostatic hypertrophy* (also abbreviated BPH) was used first to describe this condition. Histologists and pathologists, who study diseases at the cellular level, currently prefer the term *hyperplasia* to *hypertrophy*. Technically, hypertrophy indicates that the cells themselves have enlarged; however, in BPH, the cells are normal size but they have increased in number. The correct designation for this is hyperplasia. Nonetheless, the term hypertrophy is still used because the entire prostate gland itself increases in size during BPH.

In the previous chapter, I mentioned that testosterone is converted to DHT by an enzyme, 5-alpha-reductase. When the production of DHT is blocked by drugs or herbs, it often relieves some of the symptoms and can even cause the prostate to become smaller. This is the mechanism by which the drug Proscar works.

If you'll forgive a whimsical analogy, you might think of testosterone as Clark Kent and of DHT as Superman. The enzyme 5-alpha-reductase would be the phone booth where he changes. Proscar, then, is a guy in the phone booth who won't get off the phone, leaving Clark Kent stranded on the sidewalk.

The hormone DHT plays a significant role in BPH.

Saw palmetto might be playing the same role as Proscar, monopolizing the phone booth and preventing your testosterone from getting into its DHT cape. In certain studies, saw palmetto has been found to decrease, or *inhibit*, the production of DHT as well as other forms of androgens in the prostate.[2–6]

The DHT hormone binds to androgen receptors, which are protein molecules floating about within the cells. The binding might have several effects. Some experiments using cell cultures show that it causes *proliferation,* or the creation of additional cells. It has yet to be proven that this works exactly the same way in the prostate, but it's reasonable to think it might.

The DHT and the hormone receptor, now connected and "swimming" through the cell together, form a molecule with the right shape to bind to certain points along the DNA. When they do this, it switches that segment of DNA to the "on" position, allowing *transcription* to take place. The cell begins making, or increases the rate at which it is making, the proteins coded for by these sections of DNA. The new proteins will be used to build new cells, increasing the size of the prostate. Saw palmetto may also interfere with this process.

Apoptosis: Cell Population Control

DHT might not only increase cell growth in the prostate, it might decrease cell death as well. The cells that make up your body can be thought of as a population. They are "born" and they die in numbers that usually balance, so that the amount of tissue in any given organ remains about the same in a completely healthy adult. There has been some question whether the increase in cell numbers seen with BPH is a result of an increased rate of cell division, causing a higher cell "birth rate," or a result of decreased cell death rate (or both).

The type of cell death we're talking about is referred to as *apoptosis.* This process is different than when your cells die from diseases or injury. In apoptosis, the cell either dies at a time programmed by the DNA in the cell or dies in response to chemical signals it receives from its environment, like the hormone and receptor mentioned before. Apoptosis also normally occurs during human fetal development. As embryos, the webbed hands that we originally develop give rise to fingers due to the programmed death of cells between each digit.

A more useful clue that medical practitioners identified was that men can only develop BPH if they have working testes.

Scientists can track which cells are undergoing apoptosis, as well as which cells are undergoing *mitosis,* or the creation of new cells. Through experiments and observation, researchers have been able to show that, in addition to stimulating cell division, DHT in the prostate suppresses apoptosis.[7] A drug or herb that blocks DHT would therefore enhance cell death in the prostate, combating hyperplasia. I'll explain how drugs and saw palmetto may do just that in later chapters.

Androgen Receptors and DHT

Androgen receptors (ARs) could be thought of as docking sites for DHT. Unless they are present, DHT can't attach to the cell and thus has no effect. The cells of the prostate, unlike most parts of your reproductive system, continue to make ARs throughout your lifetime. This allows DHT, testosterone, and other male hormones to affect prostate tissue.

Saw palmetto might also work by blocking certain hormone receptors, thus shrinking prostate tissue.

It has been shown that the number of ARs in the nucleus of a hyperplastic prostate cell—one taken from an enlarged prostate—might be greater than in a normal prostate cell.[8] When there are more ARs present, the cell becomes more responsive to DHT, which (as we discussed earlier) could lead to increased cell production.

Some studies suggest that saw palmetto might work by blocking the ARs—rather like plugging up a keyhole with chewing gum so that the key (DHT) doesn't fit.[9] This could also lead to a reduction in prostate growth, or shrinking of the tissue. I'll go into more specifics on these findings in chapter 6.

Somewhat surprisingly, it has also been found that increased levels of estrogen might cause an increase in the number of ARs. If this is true, blocking estrogen from acting on the prostate might decrease the number of ARs, in turn reducing prostate size. This is the basis for another theory about how saw palmetto works.[10]

Embryonic Reawakening/
Cell-to-Cell Communication

In BPH your body is forming new glandular tissue. Because this is supposed to happen only when you are in the womb, the term "embryonic reawakening" is sometimes used to describe what's going on.

In normal development, the prostate cells first multiply to large numbers and then they mature. Only a mature gland cell can produce secretions—in the case of the prostate gland, prostatic fluid.

In BPH, new cells are being developed, but often there is an actual decrease in the amount of prostatic fluid produced. Something has gone awry. The cells are multiplying (when they shouldn't), but not reaching maturity. We don't know what is wrong, but some researchers have theorized that the normal communication between cells that tells them what to do has broken down.[11]

And when cells don't receive those instructions to mature, the normal process of apoptosis (automatic cell death) doesn't occur. So if the cells are receiving confusing messages telling them to multiply, but not giving them the information needed to become fully mature, your body may continue making more and more cells without having them die off at the normal rate. The end result: an increase in prostate size.

Inflammatory Cells

Special chemicals called *growth factors* (GFs), are used to control cell growth. Another theory about what causes BPH suggests that extra GFs produced by *inflammatory cells* might play a role in causing BPH by telling the cells to multiply when they shouldn't.

If We Can Walk on the Moon, Why Can't We Figure Out How Our Own Bodies Work?

S ometimes it seems absurd that with all the amazing things we have accomplished through science and technology, we don't know exactly what causes BPH. Yet the complexity of life's inner workings often thwarts our attempts to discover its secrets.

The perfect experiment has only one variable—only one thing changes. When more is occurring in a system than just what you want to study, there is doubt whether your experimental change or some random event caused the results you obtained. But each cell in your body is a complex world unto itself, constantly active, and constantly changing. Stop all those changes, and you no longer have a functional system—the cell dies.

Some biomedical researchers study whole animals, an *in vivo* study. This has the advantage of being a fully functional system, but it also has the most variables. What the animal eats, its activity level, and, for all we know, even what mood it is in can affect its biochemistry. Others use *in vitro* models, studying cells in culture (remember those high school experiments of studying cell clusters in petri dishes?). The experimenter has more control over the situation, but may lose aspects of the

Inflammatory cells, part of your body's immune system response, have been found in hyperplastic prostate tissues. If indeed the GFs are telling the cells to increase in number, then interfering with their production would slow or stop the growth of the prostate. Recent research system that are important to the experiment. Sometimes cells behave much differently when separated from the whole animal, which in itself can provide clues about what's going on. Adding one missing element at a time sometimes yields secrets about a mechanism that would be impossible to discover amid the complexity of the whole animal.

Neither the results from in vitro nor in vivo experiments can be assumed to reflect the way things work in a human being. But, together, the different perspectives offered by each method can be combined to form a more complete picture. Both of these approaches have been used in trying to discover both the causes of BPH and the mechanism by which saw palmetto can relieve the symptoms of this condition. As you will see in chapter 6, a great deal has already been learned about saw palmetto. Studying how the plant extract causes the prostate to shrink and how it relieves symptoms may someday help us to better understand the condition.

When you begin to appreciate the complexity of your own inner workings, the question that seems more appropriate than "Why don't we know?" is "How did we ever learn so much?"

published in the journal *Prostaglandins, Leukotrienes, and Essential Fatty Acids* suggests that one of saw palmetto's effects might be interfering with the production of GFs by inflammatory cells.[12] I'll discuss this more in chapter 6.

Two Types of Prostate Growth?

Either one of two different types of prostate cells can multiply and cause enlargement. One of the most confounding aspects of BPH is that it doesn't cause the same types of tissue growth in everyone who has it. In some men, the glandular tissue shows the greatest increase in volume, whereas in others the muscular tissue is more affected.

In cases in which the prostate is greatly enlarged, it has been found that most of the tissue tends to be glandular. In cases of BPH in which the prostate size is not dramatically increased, there's often a greater percentage of smooth muscle tissue enlargement.

In either case, the smooth muscle in the prostate seems to respond to the whole situation by experiencing muscle spasms. This is one of the reasons that some men with very little enlargement can still have symptoms. The contractions of the muscle tissue can cause *dynamic obstruction* of the urethra—the tissue isn't necessarily growing into the urethral duct, but the duct is still being partially closed off.

Saw palmetto might be providing relief by relaxing the lining of the urethra so that the passage is opened up.

Regrettably, perhaps, smooth muscle tissue isn't under voluntary control; you can't consciously make the muscle relax like you can with your arm muscles, for example. It has its own special brands of receptors that control tension and relaxation, one of them is called an *alpha-adrenergic* receptor. Blocking this receptor causes the smooth muscle tissue to relax. The drugs doxazosin (Cardura), terazosin (Hytrin), and tamsulosin (Flomax) all take advantage of this mechanism.

Saw palmetto has long been used as an antispasmodic, and current research verifies its effectiveness in this regard, suggesting that it relaxes smooth muscle in several ways.[13,14] Saw palmetto might be providing symptomatic relief in a way similar to the alpha-adrenergic drugs (we'll talk more about these in chapter 5), by relaxing the muscular lining of the urethra so that the passage is opened up somewhat.

In the next two chapters, which focus on the conventional treatment for BPH, I'll discuss in more detail the surgical solutions that have been relied on and how some of these theories have been used to try to find a pharmacological solution for the problem.

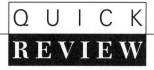

QUICK

REVIEW

- The causes of BPH are still unknown; the only factors that we know are involved include being male, being over 40 years old, and having functional testes, but we know that there's more to it than this.

- Researchers have a number of ideas about the cause of BPH, including dihydrotestosterone (DHT) causing increased cell birth and/or decreased cell death, increased ratios of estrogen to testosterone perhaps increasing the cells' sensitivity to hormones, and chemical "miscommunications" between cells that prevent the cells from maturing and dying at the proper time.

- Saw palmetto might slow down or reverse the growth of prostate tissue, and it might also relax muscle contraction around the urethra, relieving some degree of the obstruction.

Conventional Surgical Treatment for BPH

Physicians have been devising ways to bring relief to people with blockage of the urinary tract perhaps further back into time than we have written records to show. Even the ancient Egyptians used *catheterization,* or the placement of a very narrow tube inside the urethra to allow the bladder to empty. Natives of the Americas also employed this technique prior to the arrival of European settlers. This was most likely one of the earliest forms of mechanical treatment for BPH and other such conditions.[1,2]

This chapter describes the history of the mechanical means of relieving prostate enlargement, from catheters to modern surgery. Although surgical techniques have improved over the years, surgery remains traumatic. The drug and herb approaches, including saw palmetto, described in later chapters are definitely preferable when successful. However, because the history of prostate treatment begins with surgery, I'll describe these aggressive techniques first.

Early Forms of Treatment

Although it's not certain that he was really treating BPH, the sixteenth-century physician Ambroise Paré invented tools for removing obstructions of the urethra. It's possible that he was using them to treat urethral stricture, or abnormal narrowing of the urethra. These tools, referred to as *tunneling* tools, entered through the urethra itself. They were somewhat like the instruments used by today's urologists for performing a transurethral prostatectomy (also abbreviated as TURP, a process we'll talk about later in this chapter), although much more primitive and undoubtedly terribly unpleasant.[3]

Paré's methods didn't catch on, however, and until the early 1900s, the method most often used for treatment of BPH was catheterization (the same procedure used by the early Egyptians). This procedure was repeated every 6 to 12 hours to empty the bladder as needed. One man garnered himself a place in medical history by recording the number of times this procedure was performed on him—6,892![4] Repeated catheterization, however, carries with it a high risk of infection.

Other methods were also tried, with limited success. Puncturing the bladder and inserting a *cannula*, or small tube, allowed emptying of the bladder through an alternate route. Enlarging the urethra using a device similar to a balloon catheter—which is pretty much what it sounds like, an inflatable balloon attached to a tube—was done by an American doctor in 1815. Other methods attempting to enlarge the passage were invented, some with success and others without.

The discovery that removing portions of prostate tissue relieved the obstruction of the urinary tract was made by accident in 1830. A surgeon, Sir William Ferguson, in the course of removing bladder stones from one of his patients, is reported to have observed that his inadvertent removal of part of the prostate didn't harm the patient but in fact brought him greater relief. Following this experience, he incorporated the removal of overgrown tissue into his procedure whenever it seemed that it might do some good. In 1849, he formally presented his findings to his medical colleagues.

However, this method took many decades to mature. Medical science had yet to develop anesthesia and to recognize the need for sterility. Different methods of performing open prostatectomies (surgical removal of part or the entire prostate) were tried, and much debate occurred regarding which were the best, safest, and most effective. Even with the better operating conditions and increased expertise of the surgeons, the fatality rates associated with this type of surgery at the turn of the twentieth century were very high, and the search for other ways to solve the problem continued.

The discovery that removing prostate tissue relieved the obstruction of the urinary tract was made by accident.

New instruments were invented that, like Paré's tunneling tool from the 1500s, were used to remove prostate tissue from the inside of the urethra. Between the 1830s and the 1930s, an amazing number of methods and designs were used to improve the success of this operation. Some used wire loops that conducted electricity to seal off blood vessels as the surgery was performed. A couple also used water to cool and flush the area during the procedure. The cystoscope, invented in the late 1800s, was incorporated into these designs; the cystoscope's mirrors and lenses allowed surgeons to better view the procedure.

Transurethral resection of the prostate (TURP) has become the most often used treatment for symptomatic BPH.

These experiments resulted in the instruments used today to perform transurethral resections of the prostate (TURPs). In the 1930s, a system called a resectoscope was invented that continued into the 1960s to be the primary tool for this procedure. In the early 1970s, the design was improved on still further, adding fiber optics to give better lighting. Today, the addition of video imaging permits a surgeon to see the surgery being performed on a screen.

Measures of Success

To see whether treatment is working for BPH, it's useful to have a way of keeping score. Doctors and researchers have come up with several sets of questions that they use to rate how effective a therapy has been. The three assessment questionnaires most often used for documenting research are the American Urological Association Symptom Index (AUA), the International Prostate Symptom Score (IPSS), and Boyarsky's symptom score. The questions concern symptoms that you may experience but that the doctor is unable to see firsthand, such as how many times a night you need to void and specifics about how you feel. A symptom score is determined from your answers.

A person participating in a study is asked all the questions before beginning treatment and then again, often several times, during the treatment to see whether the symptom score has changed. Also, many of the same measurements used to diagnose BPH are used to track progress in studies of drugs and procedures. These include peak flow rate (PFR); the amount of urine remaining in your bladder after voiding, or postvoid residual (PVR) volume; the size of your prostate as measured by ultrasound; and prostate-specific antigen (PSA) levels.

I'll refer to these methods of measurement as we look at the surgeries and procedures available to us and how well they work. You'll see them again in the next chapter on standard drug treatments and in the chapters covering the research that has been done on the effectiveness of saw palmetto and other alternative treatments.

Surgery

The three surgical methods of treating prostate enlargement are transurethral resection of the prostate, transurethral incision of the prostate, and open prostatectomy.[5] A description of these follows, along with some information on the effectiveness and possible complications of each, so that you will be able to better compare your options.

Transurethral Resection of the Prostate

As the means for removing the obstructive portions of the prostate without having to use open surgery improved, a transurethral resection of the prostate (TURP) became the most often used treatment for symptomatic BPH. During a TURP, a surgeon passes an instrument through the urethra and removes the prostate tissue causing the blockage. Picture, if you will, inserting a tool into the core of a pear and cutting away the flesh without puncturing the pear's skin, and you have a general idea of how the surgery works. A survey done in 1986 showed that 96% of all men who had required prostate surgery had undergone a TURP. Quite likely, the other 4% had enlargement too great to allow the procedure to be done safely.

The percentage of men having TURP performed has dropped off since those figures were collected. This is probably because of the other, less invasive procedures that exist (which I'll describe later) and the new medications available.

TURP generally produces good results—better than what can be expected with drug treatment or with some of the other nonsurgical procedures. One meta-analysis in which data from several studies was combined showed an 88% chance that you would have about an 85% improvement in your symptom score.[6] This is a considerably greater benefit than what can be achieved with drugs or herbs, where an improvement of 40% is quite good.

However, surgery has its drawbacks including, of course, the discomfort, the expense, the risks, and the recovery time. There are frequently several very unpleasant days following surgery, during which you may experience painful spasms. The length of hospital stay ranges from 1 to 5 days, and the average cost in 1994 was about $7,600. That can vary a great deal, depending on what part of the country you live in, and costs have undoubtedly changed since that time.[7]

On the brighter side, when undergoing a TURP you are not risking your life. A 1994 study indicated that the mortality rate was the same for men who had undergone TURP as it was for those who had not had any surgery.[8] This is not to say that the surgery is entirely without its risks or side effects, but should you reach the point where surgery is truly necessary, it's not an unreasonable option.

The most common side effect of TURP is something called *retrograde ejaculation*. The incidence of this disorder following TURP is so high that you might just as well presume you'll have it should you have to undergo this type of surgery. It's estimated to affect anywhere from 50 to 95% of men so treated. Here's what happens: The ejaculate travels up the urethra into the bladder rather than being expelled out through the urethra. Later it is flushed out with urination. The condition doesn't prevent orgasm, but it is a cause of male infertility. A similar side effect is seen with the medication Flomax, as described in the next chapter.

About 2% of men who have a TURP experience a reaction called *transurethral resection syndrome,* which is believed to be caused by the body absorbing too much of the fluid used to flush out the tissue as it is removed. The symptoms include confusion, nausea and vomiting, elevated blood pressure, slowed heart rate, and problems with vision. The condition can be fairly easily treated and reversed, although it could increase the length of your hospital stay. This is the reason that men with very large prostates are not good candidates for TURP. The more tissue that needs to be removed, the longer it takes, and the longer it takes, the more fluid is absorbed.

Men with very large prostates are not good candidates for TURP.

Also at the 2% level is the risk of *extravasation.* This happens when the surgeon exceeds the area of tissue that should be removed and makes a hole through the capsule that surrounds it (in our earlier example, this would mean the surgeon cut too deeply and punctured the skin of the pear). The symptoms caused by this also include nausea, vomiting, and abdominal pain. The treatment generally used for extravasation is to stop surgery as soon as the puncture is noticed and insert a catheter. Your body will heal the capsule's wound, but again this could increase your time in the hospital.

With any surgery, excessive bleeding is always a risk. For prostate surgery, the risk increases for those with greater enlargement. As with the fluid absorption, the longer the surgery takes, the higher the chances of a problem with bleeding. Your best bet is a surgeon with a lot of experience and a good track record with this type of surgery.

For mild to moderate prostate enlargement, surgery may be overkill.

Earlier findings that incontinence and impotence were possible side effects of TURP have been refuted by recent studies. In a 1995 study, two groups of men with BPH were followed up after either TURP or a period of "watchful waiting" and were found to have no difference in the incidence of either incontinence or impotence.[9]

Nonetheless, for mild to moderate prostate enlargement, surgery may be overkill. Conventional medications as well as saw palmetto and other herbs like nettle root (see chapter 10) might provide relief for BPH symptoms for less money, discomfort, and risk.

Transurethral Incision of the Prostate

Very similar to the TURP method, transurethral incision of the prostate (TUIP) uses equipment that enters through the urethra to allow the surgeon to see the prostate using cystoscopy, fiber optics, and possibly video monitoring. Instead of removing the inner portion of the prostate (as done in a TURP), one or two canal-like incisions are made that open a channel in the urethra, allowing the urine to pass.

There are both some advantages and disadvantages with this method as compared to TURP. The most clear-cut advantage is that TUIP is simpler and less time-consuming. In addition, the incidence of retrograde ejaculation is greatly decreased to about 5 to 15%, depending on which study you read. There's also a reduced rate of problems with bladder neck contracture (narrowing of the neck of the bladder due to scarring from surgery), which is sometimes seen with TURP. Men who are at high risk with use of general anesthesia can have this operation with local anesthesia instead.

From the same meta-analysis that analyzed the results of TURP, there is an 80% chance that your symptom score will improve by about 73%. Otherwise, the long-term effects and complications are about the same for both methods. TUIP has been shown not to be effective in cases in which prostate enlargement is dramatic— greater than 30 ml is the most frequently used cutoff point.

For men who have symptoms but not a greatly enlarged prostate, TUIP might be worth investigating as an alternative to TURP.

The cost of a TUIP is said to be about one-sixth that of a TURP when it's performed as an outpatient procedure.[10] Some physicians perform this as inpatient surgery. Also, some physicians use general anesthesia and others prefer local anesthesia. These are considerations you would want to discuss with your doctor if you're contemplating this method of treatment.

A recent trial was done using a laser to perform a TUIP, and the results were very positive. Following surgery, both symptom score and PVR were decreased, and PFR was increased. Local anesthesia was used, and no hospitalization was necessary.[11]

Studies comparing the long-term effects of TURP and TUIP showed no statistically significant difference in symptom scores or measurable parameters after periods of about 3 to 4 years. One study did note that symptoms were increasing slowly for both groups, but 60% of the participants from both groups seemed content with the results.[12,13] For men who are experiencing symptoms but do not have a greatly enlarged prostate, especially those interested in maintaining ejaculatory function, TUIP might be worth investigating as an alternative to TURP.

Open Prostatectomy

In a very few cases, an open prostatectomy (in which an incision through the skin is made to remove all or part of the prostate) might be your only option. Extreme enlargement accompanied by severe symptoms of urinary obstruction that have not responded to other treatments might warrant such surgery. Other reasons for using this method include the presence of bladder stones that are too large to pass through the urethra, or other ailments that require lower abdominal surgery that could be done at the same time, such as hernia repair in the lower abdomen or groin region.

The recovery time for this surgery is longer than with TURP, with hospital stays ranging from 3 to 7 days, and some of the associated risks are much more serious. These include excessive bleeding, blood clots that can block blood supply to the lungs or other parts of the body (usually the lower limbs), heart attack, and stroke (see table 1). Although

Table 1. Comparison of Surgical Procedures

Procedure	Description	Cost*	Hospital Stay	Possible Side Effects	Risks
TURP	Instrument inserted into the urethra to cut away prostate tissue	$7,660	1 to 5 days	Retrograde ejaculation Bladder neck contracture	Transurethral resection syndrome Extravasation Excessive bleeding
TUIP (outpatient)	Instrument inserted into the urethra to make one or two incisions in the prostate tissue	$1,300	None	Retrograde ejaculation Bladder neck contracture	Extravasation Excessive bleeding
Prostatectomy	Removal of prostate gland (via open surgery)	$18,440	3 to 7 days	Impotence Retrograde ejaculation Bladder neck contracture Incontinence	Excessive bleeding Blood clots Heart attack Stroke Epididymitis Cystitis

* Costs may vary per location.

59

Charles's Story

C harles was a 59-year-old construction worker who had ~~thought he was in pretty good shape: reasonably low blood~~ pressure, healthy weight, and still able to put in a full day's work with the crew. But over the past year he had developed a problem that was really irksome to a guy who has to climb down a ladder every time he has to get to the bathroom. He went to see his doctor about it and learned he had benign prostatic hyperplasia.

They discussed his options. There were drugs he could try, but he was a little leery of some of the side effects, and surgery seemed a little extreme. So he chose the doctor's other suggestion, "watchful waiting," in hopes that the problem would resolve itself, as it sometimes did.

Unfortunately, it only got worse and began to interfere with his sleep, waking him up three or four times a night. So when his wife Linda came across a magazine article about something called saw palmetto, which was being used in Europe to treat BPH, he asked his doctor about it.

transfusions aren't often necessary with this surgery, some physicians recommend donating your own blood prior to the operation as a precaution. J. E. Oesterling, in *Campbell's Urology,* says, "The incidence of any one of these complications is less than 1%, and the overall mortality rate resulting from this operation approaches zero."[14]

The number of possible side effects and risks is greater with a prostatectomy than with either TURP or TUIP. Impotence following open prostatectomy is seen in 3 to 5% of patients, and retrograde ejaculation occurs in 80 to 90%.

The doctor wanted to try prescription medications first, but Charles pointed out that saw palmetto was reported to have fewer side effects than drugs (see chapter 6 for a full description of these studies). Charles showed him the article, especially the references to published studies that had been done. Reluctantly, his doctor looked into it and called Charles.

"As far as I can see from the research that's been done, it may do you some good, and it likely won't do you any harm. I guess if you really want to try it, go ahead." They scheduled a recheck for 2 months later.

It had been a surprise to the doc, Charles thought, when the stuff actually worked. His urine stream was improved. A few other little things he hadn't really noticed before had cleared up too—it didn't take him as long to start urinating, and he wasn't having that leakage afterward anymore. Better than that, the frequency and nocturia symptoms had been greatly relieved. Not entirely gone, but he made a lot fewer trips down the ladder.

Epididymitis—an inflammation of the area of the testes in which sperm are stored—or cystitis can occur as well. Symptoms of incontinence can begin (or continue) after surgery until the bladder muscles have recovered from the effects of the blockage. As with TURP, bladder neck contracture can be a problem after an open prostatectomy. The risk for any of these latter four complications is said to be 2 to 3%.

The expense is considerably greater than for TURP—about $18,440 on average in 1994, which again might have increased somewhat and will vary with location. On the basis of the types of risks involved, doctors generally don't recommend this type of surgery, unless you really have no other options.

Less Invasive Treatments

Quite a few other procedures are now available for treating BPH in addition to surgery. Some have been shown to work fairly well, whereas the reports on others are less convincing. The current list of viable nonsurgical procedures for treatment of BPH includes the following:

- Laser therapy
- Electrovaporization
- Hyperthermia and thermotherapy
- High-intensity focused ultrasound
- Transurethral needle ablation (TUNA)
- Intraurethral stents
- Balloon catheterization

Even though these procedures are less traumatic to the body, they still provide their own set of side effects. If your condition doesn't warrant surgery, saw palmetto might provide you with relief that is almost side-effect free.

Laser Therapy

Cutting the prostate tissue with a laser rather than a blade cauterizes (seals) the blood vessels at the same time, permitting a virtually bloodless operation. This can be especially important if you're taking medications to thin your blood.

Another way to use the laser instruments now available is to focus the laser beam into areas of the prostate to cause *coagulation necrosis,* in which the tissue dies because the blood supply has been closed off. This method generally requires a longer period for healing.

A third application is vaporization of the prostate tissue, in which extreme heating is used to destroy the tissue and open the urethral duct.

Laser therapy provides improvement in symptoms similar to the results of TURP. In addition to reducing blood loss, laser therapy reduces the amount of irrigation fluid absorbed compared to TURP. Either there's a very brief hospital stay or the procedure can be done as an outpatient therapy. The risk of ending up with retrograde ejaculation is also much less. This very

If your condition doesn't warrant surgery, saw palmetto might provide relief that is almost side-effect free.

promising method has been successfully tried using local anesthesia and might be an option for those at risk with general anesthesia.

Electrovaporization

Using an electrode that emits a small area of concentrated current, it's possible to vaporize the prostate tissue, similarly to the method described for laser therapy. It's the same basic process as is used for TURP: opening up a channel within the prostate. The results from studies of this method have been promising, offering shorter recovery time than with a TURP and a lower risk of problems with bleeding and absorption of irrigation fluid. The results so far seem comparable to those of TURP, but most of the authors who've published studies on electrovaporization agree that more research is needed to evaluate its long-term effectiveness.

The only drawbacks noted up to this point are that it's difficult to open as wide a channel using the electrode as is possible with the TURP and that the procedure takes longer to complete. As well (and this is true with most of the methods described in this chapter, other than TURP and open prostatectomy), tissue samples can't be taken for cancer screening.

Hyperthermia and Thermotherapy

Using heat to kill cells that are growing out of control is possible because they don't tolerate extreme temperatures as well as normal, healthy cells. Although cancer cells are the ones most sensitive to heat, the hyperplastic cells present with BPH can also be destroyed using radio-frequency waves or microwaves.

Unless your problems are sudden or acute, medical treatment with herbs or standard drugs might be preferable.

The high-frequency waves are delivered either rectally or through the urethra through a device inside a probe. The difference between hyperthermia and thermotherapy is the degree of heat—hyperthermia uses temperatures below 45°C, whereas thermotherapy uses temperatures above 45°C. (For reference, 38°C is about normal body temperature.)

Hyperthermia and thermotherapy have yielded mixed results in testing, sometimes appearing to do no more good than a placebo treatment.[15] Many of the prescribed methods are quite time-consuming, requiring the patient to come in for as many as 10 sessions, each lasting as long as an hour. Recent design changes appear to allow single sessions of about 90 minutes.

With higher-powered devices, urinary retention following treatment is a frequently occurring problem. The method is not very effective for excessively large prostates or for those in which the middle lobe is enlarged.

High-Intensity Focused Ultrasound

High-intensity focused ultrasound works on the same principles as microwave and radio-frequency waves but can also be used to heat a targeted area of tissue. Small areas within the prostate are destroyed, again causing coagulation necrosis.

Preliminary tests of this method have shown that it does improve symptoms, but there are some side effects, such as frequent short-term urinary retention and blood in both the urine and semen. Most patients need to be catheterized for about a week following this procedure.

Less-frequent side effects include urinary tract infections and epididymitis, and there were rare occurrences of injury caused by the procedure.

Transurethral Needle Ablation

Transurethral needle ablation (TUNA) also introduces radio-frequency waves into the prostatic tissue to cause cell death by coagulation. The differences between TUNA and the radio-frequency method are that needles are inserted through the urethral wall into the prostate to deliver the radio-frequency wave to a very precisely controlled location. As well, higher temperatures are used, heating the tissue to about 100°C.

At this time, several follow-up studies have been done on patients 1 to 2 years after TUNA.[16,17,18] These reports indicate that many men received good relief of symptoms with a much lower rate of ejaculatory problems. Although the symptom scores were not as universally nor quite as greatly improved as they usually are with a TURP, TUNA has the advantage of being an outpatient therapy that uses only local anesthesia with a sedative.

Intraurethral Stents

An intraurethral stent is small device that's inserted in the urethra to hold the passage open. There are several varieties. One resembles a very tiny spring. Another is a mesh, similar to very fine screen. There are even some *thermosensitive* stents that respond to the body's natural temperature, expanding to the proper size once they are fitted in place.

Stents are sometimes used when medical therapy has failed but the patient is a poor candidate for surgery. The mesh type is reported to be safer for long-term use than the spiral variety, but neither is generally intended to be permanent. Eventually, the tissues of the prostate will overgrow the stent, which must then be removed.

Balloon Catheterization

The idea of balloon catheterization is simple: to widen the urethra by applying pressure from within. The inflatable device is inserted and then inflated to a specific diameter. Overall, the results haven't been much different than those seen when patients are treated with a placebo. Although this method sounds perfectly logical, it doesn't appear to work very well in maintaining an open urethral passage.

Making Choices

All the surgical and less invasive procedures described so far involve some degree of entering the body and changing things physically. From around the 1950s until very recently, these methods have been the only ones that doctors have really used to treat BPH. Regrettably, some physicians might still see them as the first line of defense.

Unless your problems are of sudden onset and so acute that they're intolerable, medical treatment with herbs or standard drugs might be preferable, as it is gentler and less extreme. In the next chapter, I'll review the available pharmaceuticals and how they work and then, in chapter 6, compare their mechanisms of action with what's known about how saw palmetto works. Later, in chapter 10, we'll see how other alternative treatments, such as beta-sitosterol and grass pollen, might also be helpful.

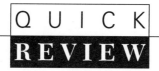

- The surgeries used in the treatment of BPH today include transurethral prostatectomy (TURP), transurethral incision of the prostate (TUIP), and open prostatectomy.
- Less invasive procedures used to relieve urethral obstruction include laser therapy, electrovaporization, hyperthermia and thermotherapy, high-intensity focused ultrasound, transurethral needle ablation (TUNA), intraurethral stents, and balloon catheterization.

- The costs and success rates of these surgeries and procedures vary considerably.
- Many physicians are still in the habit of using surgeries and procedures before trying any other treatments; however, in mild to moderate cases of BPH, drugs or herbal alternatives might be preferable forms of treatment.

Conventional Medical Treatment for BPH

I find it somewhat amusing that if you research the "conventional" approach to treatment far enough back into history, you eventually run across the sort of treatments we now consider "alternative." This appears to be the case with BPH. Some of the earliest forms of treatment for this problem were herbal. In fact, as recently as the 1940s, *Serenoa repens* was listed in the *United States Dispensatory* as a prescription for symptoms of prostate enlargement as well as bladder infections.[1]

However, this chapter will deal with those medical treatments considered to be a part of conventional medicine in the 1990s. In chapter 6, I'll cover saw palmetto and the research that has been done concerning its effectiveness and how it works.

Drug Treatments: Four Choices

The basis for the earliest attempts to treat BPH medically rather than surgically came from evidence showing that castration reduced prostate size. Researchers set about trying to create medications that could cause some of the effects of castration without the drastic measures used in the operation.

Because the testes produce androgens, the first drugs tried were designed to block the influence of such hormones. But these drugs (referred to as *antiandrogenics*) either were unsuccessful in treating the condition or caused side effects too severe to be acceptable.[2] The problem was that they didn't affect just the prostate. By blocking most of the effects of androgens, they were in many ways as bad as castration. However, this hormone-blocking method was later to resurface when more specific antiandrogens were developed, such as the drug finasteride.

Some of the earliest forms of treatment for BPH were herbal.

The second approach that was investigated for medically relieving symptoms of BPH was to reduce muscular contraction in the prostate. As with the first approach, the early attempts had mixed success, again because the drugs were not specific enough. They affected too many other parts of the body and therefore caused too many side effects.

Not until the 1990s did the FDA approve any drugs for control of BPH, but now we have four to choose from. Three of these (Hytrin, Cardura, and Flomax) are of the "muscle-relaxing" type, referred to as *alpha-adrenergic blockers*. They appear to offer quick relief, but do not actually cause the prostate to shrink. The fourth, finasteride (Proscar), interferes with a specific androgenic hormone called DHT. Proscar takes longer to work, but it shrinks the prostate and might reduce the chance that surgery will later be needed.

Although none of these drugs is as effective as surgery, they are so much less traumatic that they usually should be tried first. As we'll see in the next chapter, saw palmetto might be an even better option. In Europe, this herb is commonly the first line of treatment, and there are also other natural treatments with good evidence of effectiveness. However, because drug therapy for prostate disease is currently the standard of care in the United States, I'll first describe the available medications in some detail.

Alpha-Adrenergic Blockers

Two of the drugs used to treat BPH (Cardura and Hytrin) were initially approved for use to control high blood pressure. In the mid-1990s, the FDA approved both of them for treatment of BPH. It turned out that these medications affect both blood pressure and BPH in the same way. They block the effects of alpha-adrenergic hormones.

Adrenergic hormones such as *adrenaline* (*epinephrine* in scientific terminology) increase blood pressure. Many hormones work by locking on to a special receptacle called a receptor site. In 1947, researchers working on developing drugs for high blood pressure discovered two major types of receptors for adrenergic hormones: alpha-adrenergic and beta-adrenergic. Their functions

The basis for attempts to treat BPH medically came from evidence that castration reduced prostate size.

are slightly different, and it proved useful to develop drugs that could block either of them specifically because the more focused the effect of the drug, the fewer the side effects. Alpha-adrenergic drugs block alpha-adrenergic receptors but not beta-adrenergic receptors and are thus more specific than just an adrenergic drug.

Stimulating the alpha-adrenergic receptors increases the tension in the smooth muscles that line blood vessels and other internal parts of the body. When a drug blocks these receptors, these muscles relax, lowering blood pressure.

Hytrin, Cardura, and Flomax appear to offer quick relief, but do not actually cause the prostate to shrink.

To help you visualize "blocking a receptor," imagine this: You're planning a large meeting, but you hear that a group of protestors is planning to show up and cause, well, tension. Fortunately for you, parking is limited at the facility you plan to use, so, with all your people safely in the building, you take up as many of the parking places as you can with extra cars. Fewer spaces are available for the protestors, so their presence is limited, and there is less tension. The alpha-adrenergic blockers do the same thing—they take up all the parking spaces on the cells of your smooth muscle tissue. As we'll see in the next chapter, some researchers are investigating whether saw palmetto might work by a similar mechanism.

Hytrin and Cardura: Alpha-1 Blockers

It turns out that the prostate also contains alpha-adrenergic receptors. Specifically, it contains a type of alpha-adrenergic receptor called an alpha-1 receptor. Yes, not only does the body have alpha- and beta-adrenergic receptors, but there is more than one type of each of these. Any alpha-adrenergic blocker will relax the prostate, but an alpha-1-specific blocker is preferable because, since it is even more specific than an alpha-adrenergic blocker, it will cause fewer effects in the rest of the body. Cardura and Hytrin are two drugs that selectively block alpha-1 receptors. They cause the prostate to relax and also relax the opening of the bladder, further relieving symptoms.

But these drugs aren't completely specific for the prostate. There are alpha-1 receptors on blood vessels too, and these drugs act on them to reduce blood pressure. Of course, if you have high blood pressure, this is a good thing. But if you don't, it means that these drugs can lower blood pressure too far, a situation called hypotension (*hypo* means "too little"; *hyper* means "too much"). Because of this, the possible side effects with either of these drugs include dizziness, postural hypotension (which just means that all the blood seems to rush out of your head when you stand up, making you dizzy for a moment), and possibly fainting. Therefore, doctors usually prescribe a very small dose of either of these drugs to start out with, increasing the dose as your body has time to adjust.

Proscar takes longer to work but it shrinks the prostate and might reduce the chance that surgery will later be needed.

Fatigue is another side effect reported with both Cardura and Hytrin. In the *Physicians' Desk Reference (PDR)* listing for Hytrin, fatigue is lumped into a category called "asthenia," which also includes "weakness, tiredness, and lassitude."[3] Other adverse reactions seen in a small percentage of people taking Hytrin for BPH include drowsiness,

nasal congestion, and impotence. Cardura has been shown to cause retention of fluid (edema) and difficulty breathing (dyspnea) in some people. A study done by Fawzy and colleagues in 1995 also reported headache and nausea as potential problems. In this study, 14% of the original subjects chose to quit taking the drug because of its side effects.[4]

> **The alpha-adrenergics seem to relieve symptoms for about two-thirds of the men who try them.**

Because the drop in blood pressure really is at the root of many of these problems, researchers have been working on finding a way to relax the smooth muscle in the prostate without relaxing the blood vessels, and they seem to have found one: an alpha-1A blocker.

Flomax: An Alpha-1A Blocker

It turns out that there are different kinds of alpha-1 receptors. Yes, not only are there different kinds of adrenergic receptors (alpha and beta) and different kinds of alpha-adrenergic receptors (alpha-1 and others), there are different types of alpha-1 receptors. It reminds me of that poem by Jonathan Swift: ". . . a flea/ Has smaller fleas that on him prey;/And these have smaller still to bite 'em; /And so proceed *ad infinitum*." The one named alpha-1A predominates in the prostate but not in blood vessels.

Tamsulosin (Flomax) binds only to alpha-1A receptors. This makes it even more specific than Cardura and Hytrin.

The drug was approved by the FDA for use in treatment of BPH in April 1997. Because of its specificity, it doesn't usually lower blood pressure and has been shown not to cause the drowsiness associated with the other two medications.

But no treatment is perfect. There is one side effect that is seen with Flomax: "abnormal ejaculation." This refers mainly to retrograde ejaculation (when sperm travels upward into the bladder instead of outward)—the same problem seen as a result of transurethral prostatectomy (TURP). It was reported that 18% of the men on the maximum effective dose of Flomax experienced this side effect.

How Well Do Alpha-Adrenergics Work for BPH?

All three of the alpha-adrenergics approved for treatment of BPH seem to relieve symptoms for about two-thirds of the men who try them. A study cited in *Campbell's Urology* that tested the efficacy of Hytrin at its optimum dose (10 mg per day) reported that 69% of the participants had 30% improvement in their symptoms.[5] Cardura and Flomax have been demonstrated to have the same effectiveness as Hytrin. They are also fairly rapid in action, producing good effects in a couple of weeks.

There is one drug that has been found to reduce the chances of a need for surgery: Proscar.

We could guess at the reasons that these drugs fail to work in the other third of the population, but we would only be guessing. The reasons probably vary from person to person. The fact that one drug fails to work doesn't mean that all of them will, even in the same drug category. For example, if Hytrin fails to work, a trial of Cardura might. If both of those fail, there's still a chance that Flomax will be effective, and vice versa.

The real problem with all the drugs mentioned so far is that they only relieve the symptoms. None has been demonstrated to prevent further prostate growth. On the plus side, the manufacturers of these drugs note that prostate size has never been proven to relate to the severity of symptoms and suggest that alpha-1 adrenergic blockers still might prevent many men from needing surgery. They also point out that, in many men, the prostate stops growing on its own.

Other experts feel that because these drugs fail to prevent prostate growth, they'll prove to be only temporarily effective. They suspect that surgery will still often be necessary in the long run. Unfortunately, we don't yet know which guess is right. There is one drug that has been found to reduce the chances of a need for surgery: Proscar (finasteride).

Proscar: An Enzyme Inhibitor That Shrinks the Prostate

Finasteride (Proscar) is the drug that bases its mechanism of action on the understanding that dihydrotestosterone (DHT) is involved in prostate growth. If you'll remember, the first drugs tried for BPH blocked androgens in general. Unfortunately, they provided so many effects in the body, they weren't useful. Proscar works more selectively by just blocking the conversion of testosterone into DHT. As with the alpha-adrenergic drugs, this increased specificity has made Proscar a great improvement over earlier tries.

Pharmaceutical Treatments for BPH

Drug	Presumed Action
Hytrin and Cardura	Block alpha-1 receptors, causing the prostate as well as the opening of the bladder to relax. Can also affect blood pressure as they dilate the blood vessels.
Flomax	Blocks alpha-1A receptors, relaxing the smooth muscle of the prostate without relaxing the blood vessels.
Proscar	Interferes with conversion of testosterone to DHT, decreasing prostate size.

The FDA approved Proscar for treatment of BPH symptoms in 1992. In March 1998, based on new evidence, the FDA allowed the manufacturer to also state that Proscar can prevent the need for surgery in some men.

How Well Does Proscar Work?

In one study Proscar users showed a decrease in symptom scores of 39%, an increase in peak flow rate (PFR) of 30%, and the additional benefit of a significant reduction—18%—in prostate size.[6,7] This makes it about as effective as the alpha-adrenergic drugs. Proscar, similarly to the other drugs used for BPH treatment, seems to be effective for about two-thirds of the men who try it—but with certain conditions. Proscar only seems to be effective in men with significantly enlarged prostates: volumes of 50 ml or more. (As you might remember from school, 1 milliter is the same thing as 1 cubic centimeter.) In men without much enlargement, Proscar had been far less useful.[8,9]

Although some benefit may be seen in a month or two, full benefits require 6 to 12 months of treatment. Interestingly, because Proscar works so slowly, many physicians had come to believe that the drug was not effective and therefore seldom prescribed it. Then came a study published in February 1998 in the *New England Journal of Medicine* that showed that over 4 years Proscar reduced the need for surgery by 55%.[10] Roughly 10% of the men who took placebo required surgery during the 4-year period of the study. Taking Proscar appeared to cut this number just about in half. This result has caused some physicians to reappraise a drug that they had previously failed to appreciate.

> **Proscar seems to be effective only in men with significantly enlarged prostates.**

The study didn't show a tremendous improvement in symptom scores—only 22%, with an increase in flow rate of 17%. However, prostate volume decreased by 18% (again) in the first year and then didn't rise any further over the 4-year study period. In other words, Proscar seems to prevent the further progression of prostate enlargement. Whether this actually makes it a better treatment than the alpha-adrenergics remains to be determined. As I've mentioned, prostate size has never been shown to correlate very well with severity of symptoms.

Proscar and PSA

Another interesting, and troubling, piece of information has turned up in multiple studies on Proscar: a fall in prostate-specific antigen (PSA) levels. Men with BPH who are treated with Proscar generally show a decrease in PSA levels of about 50%.[11] This is more than can be accounted for by the decrease in prostate size, consistently at around 18%, and is a cause of great concern because PSA is used by physicians to monitor for prostate cancer. If Proscar artificially lowers PSA levels, it could prevent detection of cancer. Since prostate cancer is very curable if detected early, and PSA is one of the main screening tests for cancer, this is potentially a very serious problem.

Various complex ways of measuring PSA have been tried in order to get around this problem, such as the "free-to-total PSA" method (see chapter 2).[12] However, an article recently published in the *British Journal of Urology* states that if this special method were used, two-thirds of the cancers found in their study would have been missed.[13] So finasteride's effect on PSA seems to be a real problem.

Another proposed suggestion to solve the PSA issue is to double PSA level readings for men on Proscar.[14] The idea behind this proposal is that if the drug artificially lowers your PSA by about half, the doctor need only multiply that number by two to know what the actual level should be. However, the effect of Proscar on individual PSA levels isn't consistent, and just doubling them may lead to inaccurate results.[15] Undoubtedly,

Because Proscar artificially lowers PSA levels, it could prevent detection of cancer.

there will be more debate on this topic before it's resolved. In the meantime, a possibility of failing to detect prostate cancer is one of the risks of this drug that will simply have to be weighed against its benefits. We'll talk more about

An Alternative to Proscar

One of the senior editors of this series, Steven Bratman, M.D., shared with me the story of a new patient who came to him 3 years ago because of a bad reaction to Proscar. The man was 55 years old, looking hangdog, and feeling quite unhappy with his situation.

Although fairly young, he had developed symptomatic BPH, and his regular physician had placed him on Proscar. For this patient, Proscar was effective in treating the BPH. His symptoms were greatly diminished with use of the medication. However, he was also one of the minority for whom the drug caused unpleasant side effects—in his case, total impotence. Even so, he had continued taking the Proscar because he had been given the impression that the only other alternative available to him was surgery.

this in the next chapter, in which we review how saw palmetto may be effective without altering PSA levels.

Side Effects of Proscar

The side effects seen with Proscar are related mainly to sexual dysfunction. Remember, Proscar was developed in an attempt to imitate the biochemical effects of castration. While this goal has largely been achieved, Proscar can cause problems in line with its origin. Reported side effects include decreased libido, ejaculatory disorder, impotence, and breast enlargement. These apparently occur in a fairly small percentage of men taking the drug. In the 4-year study, the

With great pleasure, Dr. Bratman was able to inform his patient that there was another option. He prescribed saw palmetto extract at 320 mg per day. Follow-up visits with the man revealed that saw palmetto was equally effective in relieving his symptoms related to BPH and without loss of sexual function.

A recent visit to Dr. Bratman's office by this patient indicates that he's still doing great. Although this chapter focuses on conventional medical treatments, because of the great variance in individual responses to the different approaches to care for this problem, it's worth remembering that there are alternatives.

Of course, a story like this doesn't prove that saw palmetto is effective. For that, we need scientific studies as described in the next chapter.

decrease in libido and impotence was the same for the placebo group and the Proscar group after the second year.[16] However, some physicians feel that in practice the rate of complaints about impotence with Proscar is higher than would be expected from the published numbers.

This is a common occurrence in studies involving the sexual side effects of drugs: People are reluctant to report them. It takes researchers specially trained in asking the right questions to identify these problems. In chapter 6, we'll examine a study that found saw palmetto and finasteride (the generic form of Proscar) provide equal benefits—and that saw palmetto was actually associated with an improvement in sexual function rather than a worsening of it.

Costs of Drug Therapy

One of the unpleasant realities of our lives is that some-times it's not only what works best that matters—it's whether we can afford it. On the basis of the prices I was quoted locally for the drugs discussed in this chapter, I've calculated what the yearly expense for each would be. These prices, like the ones for surgery, undoubtedly vary in other parts of the country:

- Cardura, 8 mg daily: $410
- Hytrin, 10 mg daily: $539
- Proscar, 5 mg daily: $677
- Flomax, 0.8 mg daily: $920

For comparison, the yearly expense for saw palmetto could be, in some locations, as low as $180 for 320 mg per day. However, because drugs are often covered by insurance and saw palmetto is not, your out-of-pocket costs may be higher with the herb.

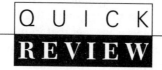

QUICK REVIEW

- Current medical therapies include alpha-adrenergic blockers (e.g., Hytrin, Cardura, and Flomax) and the antiandrogen Proscar.
- Fast-acting alpha-adrenergic drugs provide symptomatic relief, usually in a few weeks, for about two-thirds of the men who try them, but they don't stop prostate growth.

- Alpha-adrenergic drugs can cause tiredness, low blood pressure, dizziness, and fainting. Flomax does not cause these problems, but it can cause retrograde ejaculation.

- Proscar has been shown to provide about as much symptom relief as the alpha-adrenergics but works relatively slower (requiring 6 to 12 months for full effect). It is also appears to be *effective only in men with great enlargement of the prostate*, about 50 ml or greater.

- Proscar offers the unique advantage of significantly reducing prostate size and decreasing the need for surgery, but it can occasionally cause ejaculatory problems, impotence, breast-enlargement, and loss of libido.

- Another problem with Proscar is that it can reduce PSA levels, which could conceivably cause a cancer to be missed.

Saw Palmetto

The Scientific Evidence

I n chapter 1, I mentioned that saw palmetto has been well researched both in laboratories and in clinical studies. The modern use of this plant extract for treatment of BPH is *not* based on folk tales or Native American wisdom. I would denigrate neither—in fact, the original understanding of the plant's medicinal value probably did come from those sources. However, for a therapy to be recognized as having value by today's scientific community, the evidence must be more than anecdotal.

Saw palmetto is well recognized by the medical community of Europe as a safe and effective treatment for prostate enlargement. It's the most frequently prescribed treatment for mild to moderate BPH in Germany and is widely used in France, Italy, Spain, Austria, and New Zealand as well. In many of these countries, a standardized extract of saw palmetto is used as the standard against which newer remedies (such as alpha-adrenergic drugs and Proscar) are tested.

Just as with the pharmaceutical drugs discussed in the previous chapter, research on saw palmetto has included both in vitro (test tube) and in vivo (human and animal) studies. Research has been done both to investigate how the herb produces its therapeutic effect and to document that effect through clinical trials. The same standards of measurement used for the studies on pharmaceuticals and surgical outcomes have been used for these studies.

Saw palmetto is well recognized in Europe as a safe and effective treatment for prostate enlargement.

As I mentioned in chapter 4, assessment questionnaires, such as the American Urological Association Symptom Index (AUA), the International Prostate Symptom Score (IPSS), or Boyarsky's symptom score, are given to participants before, during, and after a treatment study. These cover symptoms such as nighttime voiding, urinary frequency during the day, pain or difficulty with urination (dysuria), and urgency. Changes in the symptom scores are used to monitor progress.

Additionally, objective measurements such as peak flow rate (PFR), prostate-specific antigen (PSA) levels, the amount of urine remaining in your bladder after voiding (PVR), and prostate size provide very concrete evidence of effectiveness (or lack thereof).

In this chapter, I'll first discuss the improvement obtained by patients using saw palmetto for BPH as documented by clinical testing. Then, I'll review some of the investigative studies and theories about how this plant might work. You'll learn how to properly take saw palmetto to treat BPH in the next chapter.

Clinical Studies

More than 30 clinical studies have been performed to test the effectiveness of saw palmetto in the last 15 years. Virtually all of these have yielded results showing improvements for most men in symptoms such as urinary frequency, nighttime voiding, PVR, and PFR. As well, several have documented significant reduction in prostate volume.

Saw Palmetto Versus Finasteride: Equivalent Benefits

One of the most compelling studies to date is a 6-month, double-blind, randomized, multicenter study that included 1,098 participants in all.[1] This study compared the effects of saw palmetto with finasteride (as you might recall, the generic drug name for Proscar) and found that they provided the same degree of effectiveness. The men who agreed to participate in the trial were randomly assigned to treatment with either finasteride at 5 mg daily or with a standardized extract of saw palmetto at 320 mg daily. None of the men knew which treatment they were taking, nor did any of the doctors who monitored their progress (this is what "double-blind" indicates).

In many countries, saw palmetto is the gold standard against which newer remedies are tested.

Before treatments began, all the men completed the IPSS questionnaire to obtain symptom scores as well as quality-of-life and sexual function questionnaires. Measurements were made of peak and average urinary flow rates, PVR, total amount voided, prostate volume, and PSA level. Assessments were done again at 6, 13, and 26 weeks to monitor changes.

Relief of symptoms for men in both groups was essentially identical throughout the study. For participants in both groups, the IPSS decreased 22% by the time of the first assessment at 6 weeks. By the end of the study, the IPSS for both groups was 40% lower than it had been before treatment. There was no statistical difference in symptom scores between the groups.

Fifty-three percent of the men taking saw palmetto extract stated that they felt their quality of life had improved after only 6 weeks of treatment. At 26 weeks, 69% had improvements in this category. For the finasteride group, the 6-week assessment showed that 55% of the men had improved quality of life, increasing to 73% at the 26-week assessment (see figure 4). The differences between these scores are not significant, meaning that on a mathematical

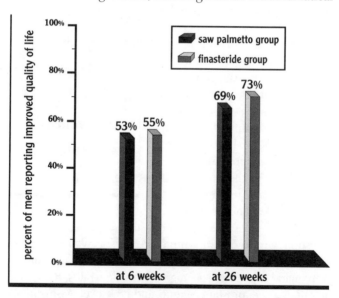

Figure 4. *Saw palmetto provided results about equal to those from finasteride.* (Carraro JC, et al. 1996)

basis both treatments were essentially identical in effectiveness. The authors of the study concluded that saw palmetto extract and finasteride were about equal in relieving symptoms of men with mild to moderate BPH.

However, saw palmetto was superior in two respects. The first was regarding sexual side effects: On average, those in the saw palmetto group indicated a 6% improvement of sexual function, whereas those in the finasteride group showed a 9% decline in their assessment scores for sexual function. Otherwise, side effects were not significantly different between the two treatments.

In a 6-month study of over 1,000 men, saw palmetto provided the same effectiveness as Proscar.

The other important difference between the two groups was the effect of treatment on PSA levels. As mentioned in chapter 5, Proscar is known to lower PSA levels significantly. In this study, finasteride caused the participants' PSA levels to drop by 41%. This is a matter of serious concern because lowering PSA levels could mask the presence of prostate cancer, allowing the disease to reach a dangerous stage before discovery. There was no change in PSA in the saw palmetto group. This is a very significant safety advantage. A doctor can recommend saw palmetto without fearing that prostate cancer will thereby be hidden.

Finasteride was better than saw palmetto in one respect. While prostate size was reduced in both groups (an important finding) the reduction with finasteride was three times greater than that seen with saw palmetto (18% versus 6%, respectively). Nevertheless, the fact that saw palmetto was found to significantly reduce prostate size to some extent suggests that it might reduce the need for surgery in the future, even if not as dramatically as Proscar. However, we can't really be sure that saw palmetto can prevent surgery without longer-term studies similar to the 4-year study completed with the medication.

While impressive, this study wasn't perfect. You may remember from the last chapter that Proscar is only effective in people with prostate sizes greater than 50 ml. To be admitted to this study, participants only had to have prostates larger than 25 ml. As it turned out, the average prostate size was just over 40 ml. Therefore, finasteride didn't have a chance to do its best. It might have outperformed saw palmetto if the men enrolled in the study had larger prostates. Also, the study only lasted 6 months, and finasteride may take 12 months to reach full effectiveness. Finally, for a variety of mathematical reasons a comparative study such as this one cannot prove a treatment effective. You really need a placebo group for comparison purposes.

Unlike Proscar, saw palmetto did not cause sexual dysfunction or affect PSA levels.

Fortunately, there have been studies that directly compared saw palmetto against placebo.

Saw Palmetto Versus Placebo

A review of published research on saw palmetto for treatment of BPH that appeared in the journal *Drugs & Aging*, examined seven double-blind placebo-controlled clinical trials of saw palmetto involving a total of almost 500 participants.[2] All but one of the trials reported significant improvements in nighttime and daytime frequency, and five showed a statistically significant increase in urinary flow. Four of the studies also reported decreases in dysuria. Although not all the investigators measured PVR, three of them did, and decreases in PVR, ranging from 15 to 50%, were seen.

One of the largest studies, conducted by Champault and colleagues, was published in the September 1984 issue of the *British Journal of Clinical Pharmacology*.[3] A total of 88 men participated, with 41 assigned to the placebo group and the other 47 taking saw palmetto extract over a period of a month. Nighttime urinary frequency was significantly reduced by 46% for saw palmetto versus 15% for placebo, and PFR was likewise significantly increased 50% for saw palmetto versus 5% for placebo. Residual urine and reports of pain with urination were also decreased by the herb.

Double-blind placebo-controlled studies of saw palmetto, involving a total of almost 500 participants, reported significant symptom improvement.

Similar results were found in a multicenter study by Cukier and colleagues, involving 146 individuals over the age of 60 with a diagnosis of BPH.[4] There was a statistically significant reduction in both nighttime and daytime urination frequency for those taking 160 mg of saw palmetto extract twice a day over a period of 2 to 3 months.

The most recent of the seven clinical trials reviewed was performed in 1995 by Descotes and colleagues, involving 176 men taking either saw palmetto or placebo over a period of 1 month (see figure 5).[5] Those who were using saw palmetto showed an overall 33% decrease in nighttime urination versus 18% for placebo, an

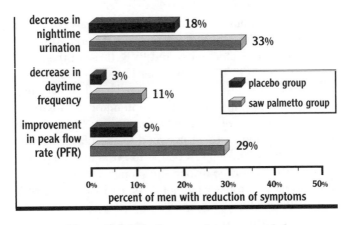

Figure 5. *Overall, saw palmetto provided more symptom relief than placebo.*
(Descotes JL, et al. 1995)

11% decrease in daytime frequency versus 3% for placebo, and a 29% increase in PFR versus 9% for placebo. All of these differences were statistically significant. The only negative side to this study was that the participants did not rate the overall effects as good enough to improve their quality of life.

Only one study did not find benefits with saw palmetto. Reece Smith and colleagues performed a trial with 33 men using saw palmetto and 37 taking placebo over a 3-month period.[6] No significant differences were seen between the two groups.

However, conflicting results are the norm in studies of any treatment, whether drug or herb. Researchers look at the evidence as a whole, and for saw palmetto the weight of the results clearly falls on the side of effectiveness.

Nonetheless, for definitive evidence of the effectiveness of saw palmetto, we really need to have a large (at least 500 participants) placebo-controlled study that lasts longer, perhaps 6 months to a year.

The Placebo Effect

Many trials of saw palmetto have been done without using a placebo; that is, study participants are given saw palmetto and the results are measured but not compared against any sort of control group. These are called "open studies" because nothing is hidden from doctor or patient. As with the double-blind trials just described, this type of study has also yielded very favorable results. However, these studies do not really prove much. The problem is the power of suggestion (placebo effect), by which people respond with improvement even when given "sugar pills."

Just how powerful is the placebo effect in BPH? In a recent study published in the *British Journal of Urology*, 303 people were given a placebo for 25 months.[7] The reported results are very interesting: Placebo treatment caused a significant improvement in symptom scores and even peak urine flow. Most of the improvement in symptom scores was seen in the first 9 months of the study, and then the symptoms began to worsen again. Even so, at the end of the 25 months, the symptom scores were still improved on average from what they had been at the beginning of placebo treatment. The peak urine flow improved throughout the length of the study. It may seem amazing that

There was a significant reduction in urinary frequency for those taking saw palmetto.

the power of suggestion can improve objective measurements like the rate of urine flow, but it can!

For this reason, you really need double-blind studies to prove a treatment effective.

Open Studies

Despite their limitations, I would like to present the results of a few studies that were not double-blind. The main reason I am discussing such studies here is to provide some evidence about changes in prostate size.

In the placebo trial just described, the participants' prostates continued to grow throughout the study, and prostate size had increased by 8.4% by the end. It appears that, although placebo treatment can reduce symptoms, it cannot stop the progression of BPH. In contrast, the evidence of several open studies suggests that saw palmetto can reduce prostate size.

I mentioned earlier in this chapter that the comparative study between saw palmetto and finasteride revealed a 6% decrease in prostate volume over 6 months' time in men assigned to the saw palmetto group.[8] Even better results were seen in an open multicenter trial of saw palmetto published in 1994.[9] With 305 participants at the end of the study, an overall decrease of 9% was seen in prostate size by day 45 of the trial. At 90 days, the average volume decrease was 10%.

In one study, saw palmetto caused a 13% decrease in prostate volume over the course of a year.

In another open trial, 42 men diagnosed with BPH took saw palmetto extract for 12 months and were evaluated before, during, and after treatment.[10] This study revealed a 13% decrease in prostate volume over the course of a year.

Because no decrease in prostate size has been attributed to the placebo effect, the result from saw palmetto warrants serious investigation. However, we need a long-term (6 months to 1 year), double-blind study that compares saw palmetto against placebo and measures prostate size to fully evaluate this subject. Even better would be a 4-year study like the one involving Proscar discussed in the last chapter, to find out whether saw palmetto can reduce the need for surgery.

How Does Saw Palmetto Work?

Because saw palmetto appears to reduce prostate size without worsening sexual function or causing changes in PSA, we can be fairly certain that it has a different mechanism of action than finasteride. However, as with most herbs and drugs, we don't know for sure just how saw palmetto works.

There are several theories about what saw palmetto does in the body. I will discuss them briefly here, but not go into great detail as in many cases the subject is rather technical.

Interfering with DHT

As you might remember, dihydrotestosterone (DHT) is believed to be at least partially responsible for the overgrowth of prostate tissue. Saw palmetto extract may interfere with DHT in a couple of ways. Evidence from test-tube experiments suggests that it may partially deactivate the enzyme that converts testosterone to DHT and also prevent DHT from locking on to androgen receptors.[11-14]

However, a study published in 1994 found that the fatty acids commonly found in the foods we eat are just as effective as saw palmetto in blocking the conversion of testosterone to DHT in test tubes.[15] This discovery raised some doubt that oral use of saw palmetto could really work by inhibiting the enzyme 5-alpha-reductase, since we would normally get a lot more of these same fatty acids from our diet than by taking saw palmetto extract.

This is a common problem with test-tube studies. Effects can frequently be made to happen in such studies that don't mean anything in real life. To better understand what saw palmetto does, experiments must be done with real people taking saw palmetto orally. Such studies have been performed, and they indicate that while saw palmetto does not appear to reduce the amount of DHT present throughout the bloodstream of men who take it, it might decrease the amount of DHT in just the prostate tissue.

In one of these studies, 32 men who didn't have BPH volunteered to be randomly placed on Proscar, saw palmetto extract, or a placebo for a week.[16] Before, during, and after this study, blood samples were taken from the men and the levels of testosterone and DHT measured. Proscar was found to significantly lower the level of DHT (52 to 60%).

However, the group taking saw palmetto did not show any significant decrease in DHT levels.

This seemed to indicate the saw palmetto was having no effect on DHT. However, a later study of men with BPH, who had been assigned to take either finasteride or saw palmetto for 3 months, showed comparable and statistically significant reductions in DHT levels in the prostate tissue specifically.[17]

As with most herbs and drugs, we don't know for sure just how saw palmetto works.

These results imply that although saw palmetto is not affecting DHT levels throughout the body, it might be having an effect that is limited to the prostate. This is all that matters after all, and if it is true it might explain why saw palmetto causes so few side effects. However, further research into this theory is needed to give any definitive answers.

Other Effects on Hormones

Numerous studies on rats and mice and in test tubes have found that saw palmetto extracts interfere with the action of other male hormones besides DHT.[18,19] Saw palmetto may also interfere with the action of various hormones deep inside the cells of the prostate. Thirty-five men suffering from BPH and already scheduled to have prostatectomies were randomly assigned to 3 months on either placebo or saw palmetto extract.[20] After surgery, tissue samples were analyzed.

The results showed that the cells had fewer receptors in the nucleus for three different hormones—various "male" hormones (androgens), plus estrogen and progesterone. Fewer receptors in the nucleus would limit the ability of hormones to affect these cells.

You may ask, what do estrogen and progesterone have to do with BPH? Good question. All the hormones in the body are interrelated, and changing one changes them all. Interestingly, the antiestrogen drug tamoxifen can relieve symptoms of BPH and also reduce prostate size to some extent. It isn't a very useful treatment, however, because in one study, 78% of the people treated with tamoxifen reported problems with sexual dysfunction.[21] Saw palmetto might provide just enough antiestrogenic effects to complement its other actions. Again, much more research remains to be done.

Saw Palmetto and Smooth Muscle Tissue

As you may recall, alpha-adrenergic blockers relieve BPH symptoms by relaxing the prostate's muscle tissue. Evidence from test-tube studies suggests that saw palmetto might have the same effect. Researchers in Italy theorized that the saw palmetto extract might be relaxing muscle tissue in a way similar to that of alpha-adrenergic blockers.[22,23] However, the evidence for this concept is still quite preliminary.

An Inflammatory Theory

The body's immune system is a complex and mysterious thing that is not well understood even now by modern medical science. Among the things that we do know is that in response to certain chemical "cries for help," your immune system will send out *inflammatory cells*. These are some of the white blood cells your doctor might look for to determine whether an infection is present in your body.

Due to recent news coverage, many physicians have heard of saw palmetto.

Inflammatory cells have been seen to invade the prostate tissue both in rats with experimentally induced BPH and in humans afflicted with the condition.[24] This invasion may be part of the cause of BPH. At least some of the inflammatory cells produce growth factors that may be sending messages to prostate cells, telling them to increase in number (as discussed in chapter 3).

A test-tube study performed by researchers in France found that extract of saw palmetto berries prevented the cells from manufacturing the chemical messenger that "requests" the inflammatory cells.[25] This could provide yet another explanation of how saw palmetto works. By interfering with the production of the chemical messenger, saw palmetto might prevent the prostate cells from receiving the calls to multiply. As you will read in chapter 10, essential fatty acids may be able to help prostate enlargement by influencing inflammation as well.

What Do We Really Know?

As you can see, quite a few theories about how saw palmetto works have been proposed and studied. We still can't claim to have one simple or certain answer. It might be that saw palmetto brings about the positive response that's seen clinically by a number of different mechanisms—in other words, it could be "all of the above."

Even drugs can have many effects at once. Plants, unlike man-made pharmaceutical chemicals, are not simply one pure compound; rather, they contain a great variety of chemical ingredients. Multiple actions are probably even more common with herbs than with drugs. Further research will be necessary before scientists can give a more definitive explanation of all the ways in which saw palmetto reduces symptoms of BPH.

What Doctors Say

Saw palmetto has been in the news enough recently so that, although many physicians might prefer not to discuss herbal remedies, most of them have at least heard of saw palmetto. James E. Powers, a doctor of pharmacology, addresses this in an article in the December 1997 issue of the *South Dakota Journal of Medicine*.[26] He seems to have written his article mainly to provide basic information on saw palmetto for doctors whose patients either are already taking it or are asking for an opinion on it. Dr. Powers comments on the fact that clinical studies have shown positive results, and that saw palmetto works without lowering PSA.

An Herbologist's Opinion on Saw Palmetto

Herbologist Susan Mead, who operates The Tree of Life, which provides medicinal herbs and consultation in Fort Collins, Colorado, has positive things to say about saw palmetto.

"There are virtually no herbs that I recommend to people just as a matter of course, but saw palmetto is an exception to that rule. I have talked to so many men who have struggled with problems with BPH. I think saw palmetto can be so helpful that I almost recommend it to all of them at a certain age."

As an herbalist whose training and background are in Chinese medicine, her approach to the use of this plant for BPH varies from that of a Western physician.

Although the author is not a practicing physician, the fact that his review of the medicinal plant appears in a journal whose audience is mainly doctors indicates that saw palmetto might be an accepted medical treatment for BPH in the very near future.

In the meantime, there are those few doctors who do incorporate herbal treatments into their practice when it seems appropriate. One such physician, Dr. Steven Bratman, has treated a number of patients using saw palmetto. He tells me that the results haven't been uniform but that he expected this to be the case.

"None of the medical treatments available for BPH work for every man who tries them. This isn't a failing of the specific drug, it just has to do with the fact that everyone with BPH is a unique individual," says Dr. Bratman. "I consider saw palmetto to be the best thing to try first, because

"Most of the work that I do is based on formulas. I very rarely will have somebody take one herb from my apothecary and utilize just that. But most of the time if somebody comes to me for enlarged prostate, I will have three parts out of eight, or even four parts out of eight, of a formula be saw palmetto. From what I've seen from the evidence, it's such an effective herb for BPH that I always like to include it."

Please note, however, that the safety and effectiveness of combination herbal treatments using saw palmetto has not been established.

it has nearly as good a track record in clinical studies as any of the other drugs on the market, providing relief without producing practically any side effects and leaving PSA alone. It also seems to work very rapidly."

Dr. Bratman gave me two examples from his practice to illustrate his point. In one case, a patient with newly diagnosed mild BPH came to him for treatment. Ralph was reluctant to take Proscar because he had problems with impotence already. Dr. Bratman had Ralph start taking a standard dose of saw palmetto, 320 mg a day. The results were quite positive. His BPH symptoms improved with no worsening of the impotence.

However, in another case, the "happy ending" couldn't be realized through drug or herbal treatment. This patient arrived at his office to discuss using saw palmetto because he had already tried both Hytrin and Proscar without success. Again, Dr. Bratman prescribed 320 mg of the herb. After several weeks, both patient and physician were forced to admit that the desired results were not being obtained, and ultimately Dr. Bratman referred this man to a urology clinic for consultation. His symptoms were relieved following a TURP.

"I don't want people to think this is a miracle cure," says Dr. Bratman, "and that's why I'm sharing this story, as well as the ones about the times that saw palmetto has worked. It's not a miracle cure any more than Proscar or Hytrin or Flomax. But it's just as good, in terms of how many people derive benefit from treatment with it. It's a viable alternative."

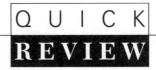

QUICK REVIEW

- A double-blind comparative study with 1,098 participants found that saw palmetto provides benefits equivalent to those of Proscar.

- Whereas Proscar caused a small decrease in sexual function on average, saw palmetto treatment caused a small increase. Otherwise, side effects were similar.

- Multiple clinical trials have shown that unlike Proscar saw palmetto doesn't lower PSA levels, which is an advantage because PSA is used as a screening test for cancer. However, Proscar shrinks the prostate more than saw palmetto, and has been proven to reduce the need for surgery.

- At least seven double-blind placebo-controlled studies, involving a total of almost 500 participants, have shown that saw palmetto extract improves both objective and subjective symptoms for most individuals.
- Several studies have documented significant reduction in prostate volume (6 to 13%) using saw palmetto.
- Although we don't know how saw palmetto works, the principal theories include interfering with the action of various hormones in the prostate, as well as antispasmodic and anti-inflammatory effects.

CHAPTER
SEVEN

How to Take
Saw Palmetto

The medicinal properties of the saw palmetto plant are contained in the berries (see figure 6). However, most people don't use whole berries or berry tea to treat BPH. You would simply have to use more berries than would be practical. Instead, virtually all the studies described in this book used a special extract of saw palmetto designed to concentrate the active ingredients. Before discussing the proper dosage and other issues, I need to explain something about these extracts.

Saw palmetto berries contain both water-soluble and fat-soluble (lipophilic) substances, but the active ingredients are contained in the fat-soluble portion. Medicinal saw palmetto products are manufactured by passing a solvent that dissolves only fat-soluble substances through finely chopped plant matter. The mixture of solvent and dissolved material is then collected and the solvent is evaporated, leaving the extract. It's similar to making tea and then allowing the water to evaporate until you have only the residue

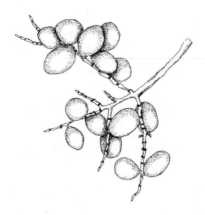

Figure 6. *The berries of the saw palmetto plant are used to make the medicinal extract.*

left in the teacup. For a standardized saw palmetto extract, all the solvents are evaporated, leaving an extract that usually contains about 90% fatty acids, plus cholesterol-like substances called plant sterols and a few other chemical "odds and ends." These odds and ends haven't been shown to be biologically active in laboratory experiments. Manufacturers usually place the extract in capsules, often (but not always) in 160-mg or 320-mg doses.

Dosage

The normally prescribed dosage is 320 mg of saw palmetto extract standardized to contain 85 to 95% fatty acids and plant sterols. According to recent research, 1 daily dose of 320 mg is just as effective as 2 doses of 160 mg each.[1] This is good news for those who have trouble remembering to take medicines more than once a day.

There doesn't seem to be any extra benefit if you take more than 320 mg of saw palmetto daily.[2]

How Much Does It Cost and Which Brand Should I Get?

Saw palmetto is widely available in pharmacies, grocery stores, and health food stores. Prices vary considerably. For standardized extract at 320 mg daily, I have seen the month's supply cost as low as $15 and as high as $30. When doing a cost comparison, don't forget to take into account what dosage each pill contains and how many pills are in the bottle. I find it easiest to look at the cost of using each product for 30 days at the recommended dosage.

Of course, cost isn't everything. If a cheap product doesn't work, the dollar savings won't help you much. On the other hand, a high price doesn't guarantee high quality either. Unfortunately, there is no good way for you as a consumer to determine if a particular saw palmetto product is worth buying. Saw palmetto is a nutritional supplement, not a drug; therefore the FDA doesn't monitor the content. There are various proposals to institute programs to impartially verify the herbal potency of supplements, but none are in place yet.

The normally prescribed dosage is 320 mg of saw palmetto extract standardized to contain 85 to 95% fatty acids and plant sterols.

Do Solvents Matter?

Three separate solvents have been used to perform the extraction of saw palmetto berries: hexane (a petroleum product), ethyl alcohol, and liquefied carbon dioxide (CO_2). Most studies have used either hexane or ethyl alcohol extracts. However, more recent studies have used extracts produced with CO_2.

Hexane is a toxic substance even in very low doses. It is for this reason that the other extraction methods have been proposed. However, hexane can be evaporated completely, leaving no residue, so safety risks are probably minimal. Ethyl alcohol is commonly used to make extracts of many herbs, and its use in saw palmetto is not controversial.

Liquefied CO_2 is a rather unusual extraction method that has recently been used with saw palmetto. You wouldn't think that a gas could be used as a solvent, but when you put carbon dioxide under enough pressure it turns into a liquid. This method is often advertised as a "nonsolvent process," but in reality liquefied CO_2 is just as much a solvent as hexane or

The best policy is to ask a health-care professional, such as a pharmacist or a physician knowledgeable in herbal medicine, for a brand recommendation. (For legal reasons, we cannot mention any brand names in this book.)

There are a number of saw palmetto products that combine other herbs, such as pygeum. If you select one of these combined products, I still recommend finding one that provides the full recommended dose of saw palmetto extract alcohol; it's just an unusual one. The liquid CO_2 is forced through the plant matter to extract the lipophilic ingredients. As soon as the temperature and pressure are returned to normal, it reverts to a gaseous state, leaving no residue.

Manufacturers can alter the temperature and pressure settings of the CO_2 extraction to affect which types of molecules will be extracted. Different settings can result in the extraction of an entirely different set of compounds. For example, one study compared extracts prepared at three different settings.[3] Although all of them significantly reduced prostate size in rats over the control group, one was found to have nearly twice as great an effect as the other two. This "fine-tuning" process may eventually result in saw palmetto extracts that are more potent than the current products. However, at present there are no studies that directly compare the newer CO_2 extracts with the old standard hexane or ethyl alcohol extracts. For this reason, we cannot say for sure which of these methods is best.

as a part of the compound. In chapter 10 we'll discuss pygeum and other alternative remedies for BPH.

When Not to Take Saw Palmetto

Good scientific evidence suggests that saw palmetto extract can relieve symptoms for men who have mild to moderate BPH. There's also documentation that it can shrink prostate tissue. However, saw palmetto is not an appropriate therapy if your symptoms of urinary obstruction are severe. Saw palmetto is not effective treatment for inability or near-inability to urinate! Severe symptoms of this type require urgent medical care.

Furthermore, make sure you really have BPH before you start self-treating with saw palmetto. Prostate cancer can cause identical symptoms, and *saw palmetto is not an appropriate treatment for prostate cancer!* Only use saw palmetto if your physician tells you that your symptoms are caused by mild to moderate BPH, and that surgery is not necessary.

What to Expect from Treatment

You can expect to notice the effects of saw palmetto in a couple of weeks, although months may be necessary for full benefit to be achieved. Typically, men report decreases in nocturia and urinary frequency, lessening of discomfort and sense of urgency, reduction in postvoid dribbling, increased stream, decreased urinary retention, and improvement in sexual function. Not all men experience all these effects, and the time it takes for any symptoms to lessen varies among individuals.

According to recent research, one daily dose of 320 mg is just as effective as two doses of 160 mg each.

A 65-year-old gentleman from the United Kingdom shared with me that after his doctor prescribed saw palmetto, he noticed a lessening of symptoms in a matter of only a week or two. He has had a decrease in general discomfort and is having to urinate at night with less frequency. Another saw palmetto user states he had a reduction in postvoid dribbling after using the herb for only 10 days and greatly reduced nocturia by the end of 2 weeks. Of course, how much of this rapid effect is due to the placebo response and how much is true effectiveness cannot be determined from such stories.

However, saw palmetto doesn't work for everyone. A 68-year-old retiree in California reports that he took saw palmetto for 6 months and that it did "absolutely nothing" for him. He found that the drug Hytrin did better. Another man reports that saw palmetto worked for about a year to relieve his symptoms, but then it stopped working. He tried both Proscar and an alpha-blocker with little success, and eventually had to get a TURP.

There doesn't seem to be any extra benefit if you take more than 320 mg of saw palmetto daily.

However, in many cases saw palmetto retains its effects for longer than a year. In one open study, men were given saw palmetto for 3 years and the improvements remained stable during that time.[4] I've heard reports from people who have been taking saw palmetto for 5 years and find it's still working. Nonetheless, since we know that placebo treatment produces long-lasting benefits in BPH too, we really need longer-term double-blind studies to know for sure how long saw palmetto keeps helping. It would also be very helpful to find out whether saw palmetto, like Proscar, can reduce the need for surgery.

Saw Palmetto and Sexual Vitality

Saw palmetto has a historical reputation as an aphrodisiac and a restorative of male sexual vitality. However, in the saw palmetto versus finasteride study described in the previous chapter only 6% of the men taking saw palmetto reported an increase in sexual function.[5] The best we can say is that the herb does not seem to impair sexual function.

How Do You Know Saw Palmetto Is Working?

We've seen the study results, but the only way to know whether saw palmetto will work for you is to try it and keep track of changes with your symptoms. Although most of the reports of success from those using saw palmetto discuss findings that physicians refer to as subjective, meaning that the doctor can't measure them, one man reports that he noticed, after a few weeks of taking saw palmetto, an increase in volume of urine output. How can he be sure of this?

"I am 58. I began noticing BPH symptoms when I was about 40 years old. I had to urinate frequently, had low volume, a weak stream, and urgency. I was generally okay at night, provided that I didn't eat anything before retiring. I might get up once during the night.

"Early on I had a cystoscopy to see what the problem was, and was told I had a moderately enlarged prostate, but nothing serious and that we would simply do 'watchful waiting' over the coming years. I was quite prepared to go on indefinitely, had it not been for the crisis caused, indirectly, by my knee surgery. I wet my pants a couple of times when I could not get to a restroom quickly enough.

"My personal physician was supportive of the use of saw palmetto, so I tried it. I know it worked because I frequently drive long distances. Over the years I found that stopping at rest stops or restaurants to urinate became a time-wasting nuisance. So I would urinate into a paper coffee cup (I drink a lot of coffee). I would pee into a 10-ounce cup and get 4 to 5 ounces of urine. After I started taking saw palmetto, I noticed that I would sometimes fill the cup, which became a problem when I was trying to drive and pee at the same time. I had to get a larger cup! Obviously, when I was able to relax and urinate at greater volumes, the number of times I had to urinate dropped."

For the benefit of future scientists conducting similar research, he also mentions that emptying the cup out the car window while driving 60 miles an hour proved "an unsatisfactory method of disposal."

A 60-year-old physician who began to have a gradual onset of symptoms of BPH almost 10 years ago has now been taking saw palmetto for 2 years and states that it works well. He mentioned that, early on when he was trying the extract, he became certain that his improvement was due to saw palmetto because he noticed his symptoms worsened if he skipped a few days. (However, this could be due to the power of suggestion as well!) He does note that some brands work better for him than others. This is not surprising, considering the lack of quality control standards. Therefore, if you try the herb without getting the results you want, you might want to switch brands. You might also want to check with a knowledgeable health-care practitioner for a brand recommendation.

Saw palmetto is not an appropriate treatment for prostate cancer!

Another man only discovered how well saw palmetto was working when he stopped taking it.

"I had been taking saw palmetto for nearly a year," chronicles a 58-year-old restaurant owner. "I didn't really expect anything dramatic to happen right away when I first started. After a couple of weeks, I thought maybe it was helping, but then for a while I wasn't sure. I just kept taking it.

After about 10 months, I just decided it wasn't doing anything for me, so I quit."

Almost immediately, symptoms that he had forgotten having had prior to starting saw palmetto returned. He found himself getting up at night to urinate—something he hadn't even noticed that he had stopped doing while taking the extract. As well, his daytime frequency increased, and his stream diminished to the point where he found he had to sit down to urinate. About 3 weeks later, he decided to return to saw palmetto therapy, and this time he noticed the difference that the extract was making.

"Now I'm certain that I'm seeing results. After 2 weeks, I was able to sleep all the way through the night for the first time in at least a month. The rest of the improvements have come back, gradually."

Although saw palmetto is the best-researched herbal treatment for BPH, other remedies you might want to try include pygeum and beta-sitosterol, which we'll discuss later. First, however, we need to talk about safety issues that relate to using saw palmetto and to review its low incidence of side effects.

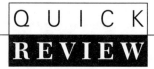

QUICK REVIEW

- Saw palmetto should be taken in the form of an extract standardized to contain 85 to 95% fatty acids and plant sterols.
- The proper dosage is 320 mg daily. You don't have to divide this up into two 160-mg doses, as a single 320-mg dose seems to be just as effective.

- Taking extra saw palmetto above 320 mg daily does not seem to provide additional benefit.

- Because of differences in manufacturing methods as well as lack of supervision by the FDA, it is quite likely that some saw palmetto products are more effective than others. I recommend consulting a knowledgeable health-care practitioner for a brand recommendation.

- Make sure to get a medical examination before self-treating with saw palmetto. Prostate cancer can cause similar symptoms, and saw palmetto is not an effective treatment for prostate cancer. Saw palmetto also should not be used for severe urinary blockage.

- For men with mild to moderate BPH, saw palmetto often provides significant relief from symptoms in a couple of weeks, although months may be necessary for full effects to develop.

Safety Issues

So, now that you've heard all about how well saw palmetto works, how well researched it is, and so on, you're braced for the bad news—the side effects. The good news is that saw palmetto causes very few side effects and is nearly nontoxic.

Saw Palmetto's Excellent Side-Effect Profile

One of the benefits of saw palmetto is that it appears to relieve many BPH symptoms without causing a lot of additional ones. The worst side effect consistently reported by saw palmetto users appears to be a mild upset stomach.

In an open study of 500 participants, only 2% of the men taking saw palmetto reported side effects during a 3-month trial.[1] In all cases, these complaints were related to stomach upset. When they took the extract with meals rather than on an empty stomach, the problem cleared up. None of the men dropped out of this study because of this symptom.

In placebo-controlled trials, only small percentages of saw palmetto users have reported side effects.[2] In six such studies, there was no significant difference in the number of side effects between those taking saw palmetto and those taking a placebo. Even in a study that showed a significant difference between the groups, the numbers were not large. Only 3.9% of the saw palmetto group reported some adverse reactions (compared to 1.1% of the placebo group). None of the reported effects were serious, and again most of them related to stomach upset.

The good news is that saw palmetto causes very few side effects and is nearly nontoxic.

Similar results have been reported in long-term studies as well. A very small percentage (1.8%) of men discontinued participation because of adverse reactions in a 3-year open study of saw palmetto; and in a 1-year open trial, no side effects at all were reported.[3,4] The only major study that reported any other side effects was the 6-month, 1,098-person trial study that compared saw palmetto to finasteride.[5] Mild elevation of blood pressure occurred in 3.3% of the saw palmetto group, and headache and back pain developed in a smaller percentage. However, it is not clear whether these effects were caused by the saw palmetto or were simply random events such as might be expected to occur in a large study. In balance, the evidence suggests that saw palmetto causes a very low incidence of side effects.

Toxicity

Toxicity is a somewhat different issue from side effects. The term primarily refers to death or serious injury caused by one-time exposure to a high dose of a substance, or lower doses over a long period of time. Saw palmetto seems to possess very little if any toxicity.

In studies during which animals were fed 22 times the equivalent of a standard human dose of saw palmetto extract, the animals displayed no signs of toxicity or changes to DNA.[6] In long-term human trials of saw palmetto, no toxic effects have been observed.[7]

Drug Interactions

There are no known drug interactions with saw palmetto.[8]

Who Shouldn't Take Saw Palmetto?

With many drugs and herbs, there are certain situations in which the treatment should not be used. These are called contraindications. For example, people with a bleeding disorder should not take ginkgo, because ginkgo may worsen the condition. However, according to the Commission E Monograph, there are no known contraindications to the use of saw palmetto.[9] These monographs are more or less the equivalent of the *Physicians' Desk Reference (PDR)* for plant medicines in Germany and represent the cumulative German medical experience with herbal medicines.

Only 2% of the men taking saw palmetto reported side effects during a 3-month trial.

However, there is one potential risk with saw palmetto. Because the symptoms of BPH and of prostate cancer are

Harold's Story

Harold was 68 years old, nearing retirement as a real estate broker. He'd been diagnosed with BPH a few years earlier, but he hadn't experienced any obvious symptoms. Then, he noticed it was taking him longer to urinate, and he was needing to get up a few times to relieve himself most nights.

After seeing a TV program about an herbal medicine called saw palmetto, Harold was thinking that maybe he should try it. Since he already knew that he had BPH, maybe he could save some money, and avoid the dreaded rubber-glove exam.

He decided he should find out more about the plant first, though. Harold turned to the Internet for information. A few abstracts on Medline and a fairly extensive Web site told him what he needed to know: The plant appeared to be at least as effective for BPH as some of the pharmaceutical drugs out there—but treating himself without seeing his doctor first wasn't a good idea. He called his physician and scheduled an appointment.

identical, it would be easy to mistake one for the other. Fortunately, this is a risk that you can avoid entirely and very simply. Just go see your doctor for a diagnosis first. If, as in most cases, your symptoms are caused by BPH, you'll know that saw palmetto is an alternative that you could benefit from.

The PSA Controversy

One of the benefits of saw palmetto in regards to prostate cancer is that saw palmetto does not appear to lower prostate-specific antigen (PSA) levels—high levels of which are

Believing the exam to be a routine precaution, Harold was shocked when his biopsy was positive for prostate cancer. He hadn't even thought about that possibility.

The urologist recommended surgery, and Harold's doctor agreed that this was the wisest course of action.

Five years later, Harold is still going strong. There is no sign of any cancer recurrence, and his doctor feels that he no longer even has to worry about it coming back. Harold was very lucky that he did not simply take saw palmetto instead of visiting his doctor. It's quite possible the herb might have relieved his symptoms while the cancer continued to grow. Even a few months' delay might have allowed the cancer to reach a stage where it was no longer curable.

The bottom line: See a physician to make sure you have BPH before self-treating with saw palmetto.

considered an indication of cancer.[10] Since the drug Proscar does lower PSA levels, in this regard saw palmetto is actually a safer choice. As you might recall from chapter 2, if saw palmetto lowered PSA, this could cover up the detection of prostate cancer.

Unfortunately, there have been several incorrect statements made in various publications and on the Internet that saw palmetto extract lowers PSA. Despite this widely repeated rumor, there is not, and never has been, any documentation from clinical trials of saw palmetto that support this claim. In fact, evidence from several studies shows that saw palmetto doesn't lower PSA.[11,12]

A Dangerous Misunderstanding: Saw Palmetto and Prostate Cancer

Not only do some people falsely believe that saw palmetto reliably lowers PSA levels, a couple of authorities at least have made a dangerous conclusion from this incorrect information: that saw palmetto can be used to treat prostate cancer.

One physician states that he doesn't rush his patients off for a biopsy in response to their having an elevated PSA.[13] Instead, he encourages a low-fat diet and prescribes 360 mg of saw palmetto extract per day as well as zinc and some antioxidant vitamins and minerals. Then he rechecks the patient's PSA level periodically. This physician claims that often the PSA level drops with this treatment plan.

There are no known contraindications to the use of saw palmetto.

This whole approach is mixed up. First, the evidence from research studies clearly shows that saw palmetto will *not* lower your PSA. Second, there's no reason to believe that just because a treatment lowers PSA levels it means that prostate cancer is being cured. After all, Proscar reliably lowers PSA, but no one is seriously saying that it cures prostate cancer. The PSA level is only a screening tool used to look for signs of prostate cancer. Believing that you can control cancer by reducing PSA is like thinking you can slow down your car by breaking the plastic on your speedometer and pushing down the needle.

If your doctor finds that your PSA level is inordinately high, delaying or avoiding a biopsy could prove fatal. Given that there's a 100%, 5-year survival rate for prostate cancer using conventional therapies before the cancer spreads, I would not want those near and dear to me to think saw palmetto would cure their cancer without some genuine evidence to support such an idea. And there is no such evidence. (For more information on cancer, see *The Natural Pharmacist Guide to Reducing Cancer Risk.*)

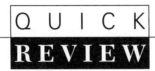

- Saw palmetto appears to be a very safe treatment.
- In animal studies, 22 times the equivalent of a normal human dose did not cause any noticeable harm, and no significant problems have been seen in long-term human studies of saw palmetto either.
- Saw palmetto's only well-documented side effect is occasional mild gastrointestinal upset, which seems to be relieved in most cases by taking the extract with food.
- There are no known contraindications or drug interactions with saw palmetto.
- The most critical safety issue is to see your doctor about your symptoms to make certain they are due to BPH and not prostate cancer, for which saw palmetto is not effective.
- Evidence from clinical trials clearly shows that saw palmetto actually offers an extra safety factor over finasteride by not altering PSA levels; thus, saw palmetto won't hide cancer from detection.

CHAPTER
NINE

How Saw Palmetto Compares with Conventional Medications

For many years, conventional treatment of BPH consisted of surgery. Only within the last decade have there been any good pharmaceutical alternatives. But choosing amongst all of your options can be quite a task. Alpha-blocker drugs (Cardura, Hytrin, and Flomax) have been shown to be effective in treating BPH symptoms, and finasteride (Proscar) can decrease prostate size, but each of these useful treatments has its drawbacks. Saw palmetto appears to be a very viable option in all cases when surgery is not necessary. This chapter discusses the pros and cons of each treatment in order to help you make an informed decision.

There are many points to consider. For example, Hytrin and Cardura give quick relief from symptoms, but they can cause quite a few side effects and, unlike Proscar, they might not help avoid surgery. Proscar causes few side effects, but it takes many months to work and may interfere with cancer screening by artificially lowering PSA levels. Flomax may be helpful for those who become dizzy or faint using

Cardura or Hytrin, but it causes its own side effects, most notably ejaculation problems.

In comparison, saw palmetto has shown symptomatic benefits at least as good as those of Proscar, without serious side effects and without lowering PSA levels. Saw palmetto has also been shown to significantly reduce prostate size. However, we don't know whether saw palmetto can reduce the need for surgery like Proscar can. Decisions, decisions. Life seldom makes important decisions easy.

Choosing the Right Treatment for You

When selecting a treatment, you are probably most concerned about what will work the best. However, as I've

noted, not everyone responds to the same medications. What works for one person might fail for another. What we can say in general is that all the treatments mentioned here, both the pharmaceuticals and saw palmetto, seem to work for about two-thirds (66%) of the men who try them. To some extent, then, finding the right therapy for you is a matter of trying them out and seeing whether they work.

Saw palmetto has been shown to provide relief equivalent to that from Proscar.

If saw palmetto is effective for you, I don't recommend adding another medication on top of the herb. There is no evidence that it will give you any added benefit, and we don't know anything about the safety of such combinations.

If saw palmetto does not work, however, there's no point in continuing to take it. You can consider trying one of the other herb and nutritional supplement treatments described in the next chapter. You can also try using one of the available medications.

In deciding whether to start with a drug or saw palmetto, the following points need to be considered:

- How promptly relief is obtained
- Benefits (in this case, a balance between long-term and immediate ones)
- Side effects
- Cost

How Much Relief, How Soon?

For the alpha-adrenergics (Hytrin, Cardura, and Flomax), about two-thirds of men using them show 30% or more improvement of their symptoms. For example, as we saw in chapter 5, flow rates increased by 30% or greater in slightly more than half the individuals using these medicines.

It takes around 2 to 4 weeks to begin seeing the effects of any of these three drugs. If you've been using them for 6 weeks or more and haven't felt any improvement, it might be time to try another remedy.

Although they provide quick relief, none of the alpha-adrenergic blockers causes a decrease in prostate size, so long-term benefits are questionable.

Alpha-adrenergic blockers provide quick relief but do not decrease prostate size, so long-term benefits are questionable.

The big potential advantage of the drug Proscar is that in a recent study (detailed in chapter 5) it was found to decrease by 50% the number of men who required surgery after 4 years of treatment. This is presumably due to its ability to significantly shrink the size of the prostate.

Unfortunately, Proscar appears to be effective in relieving symptoms of BPH *only when prostate size is 50 ml or greater.* Remember, a very large prostate does not indicate worse BPH. It's simply that some men with BPH have larger prostates than others, and Proscar only works in those whose prostates are at the large end of the scale. In those with prostate sizes greater than 50 ml, Proscar appears to be approximately as effective as alpha-adrenergics. However, it works more slowly, taking 6 months to a year to achieve full effect. Some benefits are usually seen in a couple of months.

Proscar was found to decrease by 50% the number of men who required surgery after 4 years of treatment.

Saw palmetto has been shown to provide relief from symptoms of BPH equivalent to that from Proscar.[1] The herb also appears to reduce prostate size, although not to the same extent as Proscar. It's possible (but not yet proven) that the long-term benefits of Proscar, which are presumed to be due to the reduction in prostate size, might be available with saw palmetto. However, because saw palmetto doesn't shrink prostate tissue as much as Proscar, it might not decrease the need for surgery as dramatically, if at all. Direct evidence from long-term studies is lacking.

It is also widely believed that saw palmetto has a more rapid onset of action than Proscar, but this has not been proven. In the major comparative study of 1,098 men (discussed in chapter 6), the two treatments were working equally well at the first checkpoint (6 weeks).

Side-Effect Comparison

The hope of lower side effects is one reason people look to herbs instead of drugs. Saw palmetto does have an excellent side-effect profile, seldom causing any problem other than mild stomach upset, and even that occurs rarely. The reported incidences of side effects with Hytrin and Cardura are also quite low. However, the types of side effects seen are more serious. One of these side effects, fainting, can carry with it a degree of risk for serious injury, particularly in older gentlemen. Other side effects seen with these drugs include dizziness, headaches, and fatigue.

Saw palmetto seldom causes any problem other than mild stomach upset, and even that occurs rarely.

Flomax, an alpha-adrenergic blocker that's designed to relax the urethra without affecting blood pressure, does not cause fainting. However, up to 18% of men using Flomax report retrograde ejaculation, a side effect that can interfere with sexual pleasure.[2]

Studies of Proscar have reported very few side effects. In the major comparison trial with saw palmetto described in chapter 5, the drug was not associated with any more side effects than saw palmetto.[3] However, participants' sexual function self-evaluations found that Proscar led to a net 9% decrease in sexual capacity, while saw palmetto

Which Treatment to Use?

A retired gentleman, who was willing to share his history, tells me that he was placed on Flomax after Proscar failed to have any effect on his BPH symptoms.

"I was on Proscar for 4 months and didn't see any improvement. A new urologist told me it was not an appropriate drug for my condition."

Since Proscar didn't seem to be working, the new urologist probably concluded that the prostate was not greatly enlarged—Proscar is usually most effective when enlargement is fairly extreme. It's also possible that he had not responded to Proscar because he had not waited long enough. Proscar's effects are sometimes not seen for 6 months. In any case, the new doctor placed him on Flomax.

About the Flomax, he says, "I didn't like it. There were no noticeable improvements, and besides that, it gave me a stuffy nose—which wasn't listed on the package warnings as a side effect. It also caused retrograde ejaculation, which was quite unpleasant!" Using saw palmetto might have been a better choice for this gentleman. There is a good chance he could have found relief for his symptoms without those side effects.

was associated with an average 6% improvement. This agrees with the impression of many physicians who feel that Proscar impairs sexuality more frequently than is reported in the literature. One family practitioner I spoke with said that, from his personal observations, he felt the rate of impotency associated with use of Proscar was closer to 25%.

As noted in chapter 5, you really need a specially trained interviewer to identify the sexual side effects of medications. Thus far, studies of Proscar have not reported taking such extra steps to get information men may be reluctant to confess. Until this is done, questions will remain about the sexual side effects of this very useful drug.

The greatest problem with Proscar appears to be that it disproportionately lowers PSA levels, the one most effective tool available for detecting prostate cancer. If measurements of PSA levels are not accurate because they've been artificially lowered by Proscar, doctors may overlook possible prostate cancer. Saw palmetto doesn't present this risk.

The greatest danger with Proscar is that it disproportionately lowers PSA levels. Saw palmetto doesn't present this risk.

Cost Comparison

As mentioned in chapter 7, there are several different forms of saw palmetto and many different manufacturers of each form. Therefore, the cost of saw palmetto can vary greatly. In stores in my area, the least expensive brand cost $15 for a month's supply of standardized extract.

I also called several local drugstores, and the lowest prices for the pharmaceuticals were $45 per month for Hytrin, $34 per month for Cardura, $76 per month for Flomax, and $56 per month for Proscar (see table 2). However, if your medication is covered by insurance, it may cost you less out of pocket than saw palmetto.

Table 2. Cost Comparison of Saw Palmetto and Pharmaceuticals for BPH

Therapy	Approximate Monthly Cost
Saw palmetto	$15 to $30
Cardura	$34
Hytrin	$45
Proscar	$56
Flomax	$76

Making the Decision

In Germany, herbs are more commonly used for BPH than any other options, and saw palmetto is one of the most

commonly used herbs.[4] Saw palmetto certainly appears to be a logical first choice, as it appears to be as effective as standard medications, costs less money, and produces fewer and less serious side effects. Its only disadvantage is that, unlike Proscar (but like all other medical treatments for BPH), it has not been shown to reduce the need for surgery. However, the effectiveness of Proscar appears to be limited to men with significantly enlarged prostates, and it may mask prostate cancer by lowering PSA levels.

The reported incidences of side effects with Hytrin and Cardura are low. However, the types of side effects seen are more serious.

The best way to decide what treatment to take is to discuss all the pros and cons with your physician.

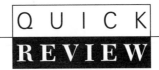

- Saw palmetto appears to be about as effective for BPH as standard medications, but it causes fewer and milder side effects (mainly stomach upset).

- Saw palmetto costs significantly less than any conventional medication.

- The drug Proscar has been shown to reduce the need for surgery, but we do not know whether saw palmetto provides the same benefit.

- The problem with Proscar is that it appears to work only in men with quite large prostates (greater than 50 ml), and it may mask prostate cancer.

- The ultimate decision as to what treatment is best for you should be made in consultation with your physician.

Other Alternative
Treatments for BPH

Besides saw palmetto, there are a number of other plant-derived treatments for BPH. Some have been fairly well researched. For all of them, there have been at least a few studies. We'll discuss what evidence there is to support the efficacy of each in the following sections.

In addition to considering medication or herbal treatments for BPH, it may also be beneficial to take a look at your whole self—what you eat, how you live, whether you exercise, and so on. We don't know exactly how your lifestyle affects the health of your prostate. However, it's generally true that taking good care of your mind and body will benefit all of your parts.

Other Remedies from Nature

It's sometimes difficult to find herbal medicines that have been well researched and found to be effective for a given ailment. However, men with BPH can choose from among a number of possibilities. We'll see that several herbal treatments for prostate enlargement that have pretty good science behind them. Though saw palmetto appears to be the best-researched herbal remedy for this condition, pygeum, nettle root, grass pollen, and others have been studied with encouraging results.

Pygeum africanus: First Runner–Up to Saw Palmetto, But It's Endangered

The tree *Pygeum africanus* is found in central and southern Africa. Although it's an evergreen, it's a very tall,

broad-leaved tree with bark that appears to have crevices up and down the length of its trunk. The native people there have used this tree for centuries for healing purposes to treat bladder pain and urinary problems, mixing a dust-like powder of the bark with milk.

There are several herbal treatments for prostate enlargement that have pretty good science behind them.

What Is the Scientific Evidence for Pygeum?

Pygeum has been studied almost as well as saw palmetto, and in some respects its research record is even better. At least nine double-blind trials of pygeum versus placebo have been performed, involving a total of over 600 participants, and ranging in length from 45 to 60 days.[1] This is a larger body of evidence than the double-blind placebo-controlled studies of saw palmetto. However, pygeum has no study equivalent to the 1,098-person study that compared saw palmetto to the drug Proscar.

The largest study of pygeum enrolled 263 individuals, given 100 mg a day of pygeum bark extract for a period of 60 days. Researchers found that pygeum can produce significant relief of BPH symptoms, including pain with urination, frequency, nighttime voiding, flow rate, and urinary volume.

Although there is much we still don't know, pygeum is believed to work by influencing the secretory cells in the prostate and seminal vesicles and also by reducing inflammation. It is not clear from the study results just how much pygeum can reduce prostate size on average, but various studies of pygeum report that unspecified prostate size reduction was seen in some participants.

Interestingly, one study found saw palmetto to be slightly more effective than pygeum for relief of BPH symptoms. For this reason, as well as the fact that the

Double-blind trials of pygeum versus placebo have been performed, involving a total of over 600 participants, and ranging from 45 to 60 days.

pygeum tree has become somewhat endangered by overharvesting, saw palmetto is probably a better first choice. (For more information on pygeum, see *The Natural Pharmacist: Your Complete Guide to Herbs.*)

Dosage

An appropriate dosage of pygeum is 100 to 200 mg daily, usually given in two doses. I recommend using a standardized extract that contains 14% triterpenes and 0.5% n-docosanol, because that is the most studied form of pygeum. Some manufacturers combine pygeum with other

Popular Herbs in Europe

In Germany, herbs are by far the predominant treatment for BPH. A new drug must prove that it is better than existing herbal treatments to be accepted! In 1995, the most widely used plant medication for BPH was beta-sitosterol extracted from the herb *Hypoxis rooperi.* The next most popular was saw palmetto, and after that came nettle. Pygeum is not used in Germany, but it is well accepted in France and Italy.

herbs used in the treatment of BPH (such as nettle) and a lower dosage of pygeum may be effective in such combinations (see Nettle Root).

Safety Issues
Toxicity studies and clinical studies haven't revealed any serious adverse effects from pygeum. Mild stomach upset seems to be the most common complaint.[2]

Nettle Root: Works Well with Pygeum
Nettle—a plant whose touch can raise burning welts on the skin—can also act as a medicine for certain ailments. The plant has dark-green leaves with serrate edges and usually ranges from 2 to 3 feet in height. It grows worldwide in uncultivated spaces. Historically, the leaves of this plant have been used to treat bites, stings, joint ailments, lung disorders, and fluid retention and were reported to be of benefit during pregnancy, childbirth, and nursing.

The leaves are also known for their food value, providing many vitamins and minerals as well as high-quality protein.[3] Once dried or steamed, the leaves no longer act as a skin irritant. The roots were found to have value for treatment of BPH by researchers in the late 1970s.

What Is the Scientific Evidence for Nettle Root?

Nettle root has not been as thoroughly researched as saw palmetto or pygeum, but some investigative research and several clinical studies have been performed.

The results of one double-blind placebo-controlled trial involving 50 participants found a 44% increase in the volume of urine produced using 600 mg of extract daily for a 9-week period.[4] Another double-blind placebo-controlled trial followed 40 men given either placebo or 1,200 mg of nettle extract over a 6-month period. Participants in the treatment group showed a significant decrease in frequency of urination.

Other studies, both open and placebo-controlled, have found improvements in symptoms such as those mentioned here as well as a lessening of nocturia, flow rate, and postvoid residual (PVR) urine. Two open studies found decreases in prostate size, although the average quantity of this decrease has not been properly reported.

We don't really know how nettle works. However, it appears to interfere with sex hormone–binding globulin (SHBG), and this might produce benefits in BPH for reasons that are too complicated to explain here.

Nettle root is listed by Germany's Commission E for treatment of urination difficulties resulting from mild to moderate BPH.

Nettle root extract might also bind to the cell membranes of prostatic cells and prevent them from dividing to create more cells. (For more information on nettle root, see *The Natural Pharmacist: Your Complete Guide to Herbs.*)

Dosage

Nettle root is listed by Germany's Commission E and the European Scientific Cooperative on Phytotherapy (ESCOP) as having medicinal value for treatment of urination difficulties resulting from mild to moderate BPH. The recommended dosage is 4 to 6 g daily of the whole root (used to make tea) or 600 to 1,200 mg of nettle root extract daily.

Studies indicate that using nettle root in combination with pygeum may be more effective than using either extract alone.[5,6] It may be possible to use half the normal dose of each and achieve equal benefits.

Safety Issues

Side effects with the use of nettle root extract appear to be rare. Of the few individuals reporting adverse reactions, most of these mention mild stomach upset. Even less frequently seen are cases of skin rashes or excessive perspiration. In a study reviewed in the book *Rational Phytotherapy*, of 4,087 people using nettle root extract over a 6-month period, fewer than 1% reported any side effects.[7] In Germany, where nettle root is widely used, the herb is believed to be quite safe. However, extensive formal safety studies have not been performed.

No drug interactions or toxicity from overdose have been reported.[8] It has been suggested that nettles should not be combined with sedatives or with medications used to treat diabetes or high blood pressure, but these comments apply to the leaf and not the root.

Grass Pollen: A Common European Treatment Not Widely Available in the United States

A grass pollen extract made primarily from rye pollen has shown some fairly promising results in treating BPH. Germany's Commission E has listed the product as useful for urinary symptoms related to BPH. The approved preparation also contains extracts from timothy pollen and corn pollen.

What Is the Scientific Evidence for Grass Pollen?

Grass pollen extract has been found in a few clinical trials to be effective in treating BPH. In a double-blind study, 60 individuals were assigned to either 92 mg of grass pollen extract or placebo for a 6-month period.[9] Sixty-nine percent of the participants using the grass pollen extract reported improvement of their symptoms versus only 30% of those taking a placebo. Residual urine was also reduced.

Sixty-nine percent of the participants using grass pollen extract reported improvements in their symptoms.

An earlier trial, also double-blind and placebo-controlled, found that men in the treatment group had significant reduction in nocturia and residual urine volume as compared with placebo.[10] Neither trial resulted in significant improvements of urine flow or voided volumes, although some of the open and comparative studies have reported increased flow rates. Good results have also been seen in two other studies.[11,12]

Although we don't really know how grass pollen extract works, researchers suggest that it might inhibit both prostate inflammation and tissue growth. Rumors that grass pollen can treat prostate cancer are based only on test-tube studies and can't be regarded as well founded.

Safety Issues

No serious side effects have been noted using grass pollen extract. As usual, a few people enrolled in studies have reported mild stomach upset and skin rashes.

While comprehensive safety studies of grass pollen extract have not been completed, grass pollen is believed to be safe.[13] However, if you know that you are allergic or extremely sensitive to the sources of the pollen used in the extract, you might want to avoid this remedy.

Beta-Sitosterol: Very Popular in Europe, But Not Widely Available in the United States

Beta-sitosterol is a plant sterol found in quite a few of the plants known to be useful in treating BPH. A particular plant found in southern Africa, *Hypoxis rooperi,* contains high levels of beta-sitosterol and is used as a source for a relatively pure extract that is the most popular herbal treatment for BPH in Germany. I say "relatively" because, although only the portion of the extract that contains beta-sitosterol is used, other components are present, some of which are also thought to be active ingredients, such as beta-sitosterolin.

An extract containing beta-sitosterol is the most popular herbal BPH treatment in Germany.

Despite its great popularity in Germany, there haven't been as many studies done on beta-sitosterol as on the other alternative treatments we have discussed here. However, those few that have been done support the idea that beta-sitosterol can provide some relief from symptoms of BPH.

A double-blind placebo-controlled clinical trial of beta-sitosterol using 200 men with BPH showed improvement in symptoms as well as increased flow and decreased PVR volume.[14] The differences seen were statistically significant compared with the placebo group. However, no change in prostate size occurred after 6 months of treatment. No side effects were reported in this study. Other placebo-controlled studies have shown similar results.[15]

Although we don't know for certain how beta-sitosterol works in BPH, it has been found to bind to tissue in the prostate and apparently affects prostaglandin metabolism.

The typical dosage of beta-sitosterols is 60 to 130 mg daily. The evidence of animal and human studies suggest that beta-sitosterol is quite safe.

Pumpkin Seed: Seems to Lower DHT Levels

Pumpkin seeds have been used for medicinal purposes in countries from Turkey to Peru for centuries. In folklore, they have been recommended for urinary symptoms and a number of other conditions.

Practically no research has been performed to confirm the effectiveness of pumpkin seeds for treatment of BPH; however, some data have been gathered regarding the soft-shelled varieties. A study that used cells in culture showed that certain plant sterols found in the seeds separate DHT from the receptors it was bound to (DHT has been implicated in BPH, as described in chapter 2). A very limited clinical study that included six men who had been scheduled for prostatectomy supports those findings.[16] After 2 days, the men who took 90 mg of a pumpkin seed extract containing only the sterol portion had much lower levels of DHT than men who hadn't used the seed extract. However, this study was far too small to mean much, and in any case it did not evaluate improvements in the symptoms of BPH.

Pumpkin seeds are often eaten whole or are ground to a powder, although oil from the seeds and extracts are sometimes used as well. Manufacturers sometimes include pumpkin seed or a derivative of pumpkin seed in combination with other herbs used for BPH treatment. Germany's Commission E recommends a dosage of 10 g of ground pumpkin seeds for the indication of urinary symptoms related to BPH.[17]

Nutritional Supplement Treatments for BPH

Other nutritional supplements that have been used in the treatment of BPH include zinc; a combination of amino acids that includes l-glutamic acid, l-alanine, and glycine; and essential fatty acids.

Zinc: Wait for More Research

Although a number of laboratory studies have offered some theories about the mechanisms by which zinc might be effective as a treatment for BPH, very little in the way of clinical studies has been done to verify them. One open study, reported informally at a conference in Chicago in 1974, showed favorable results for 19 individuals taking 150 mg of zinc for 2 months, followed by a reduced dosage of 50 to 100 mg daily.[18] All participants claimed to have an improvement of their symptoms, and 14 of the 19 were seen to have decreases in prostate size. However, because we know that placebo treatment can dramatically improve prostate symptoms, these results can't be taken as particularly meaningful. On the other hand, the observed reduction in prostate size might be significant, since shrinkage of prostate tissue has never been shown to be an effect of placebo treatment in BPH. Nonetheless, until zinc is shown to work in double-blind trials, its effectiveness in BPH must be regarded as completely unproven.

Despite this lack of evidence, many practitioners (including some urologists) recommend zinc for prostate problems, most often as a supplement in combination with some other medical therapy. The recommended dosage of zinc is 30 mg daily. It should be combined with 1 to 3 mg of copper daily, as zinc interferes with copper absorption. Don't exceed this dosage except on a physician's advice. Zinc is toxic when taken in excess.

Pumpkin seeds have been used for medicinal purposes in countries from Turkey to Peru for centuries.

Amino Acids: A Promising Option That Seems to Have Been Forgotten

Amino acids are the pieces that make up proteins. Our bodies make proteins constantly—to replace old cells, to create the secretions that we need to function, to add muscle tissue when we have been exercising, and so on. Twenty amino acids are needed for the body to remain healthy. Eleven of these our systems can create for themselves, if we haven't consumed any recently, by dismantling others and then using the "spare parts." These are referred to as *nonessential amino acids.*

A few older scientific studies suggest that the nonessential amino acids L-glutamic acid, L-alanine, and glycine, when taken in combination may relieve symptoms of BPH and reduce prostate size. A study published in 1962 included 85 participants.[19] Forty of these were given placebo, and

Combining Therapies

As we've seen in the clinical trials of saw palmetto and other treatments in this book, herbal medicines can be a powerful part of your health-care program. A few studies have been done on combining various herbal medicines, such as pygeum and nettle root, and many manufacturers combine multiple alternative remedies into one pill. However, the effectiveness of combinations containing numerous herbs has not been scientifically proven. Treatments that offer certain benefits when used alone do not necessarily produce even greater benefits when combined. They can just as easily interfere with each other. To use the analogy of a previous chapter (and slightly distort comic book lore), if Bruce Wayne and Clark Kent both rush toward a certain telephone booth at the same instant, it could happen that they get in each other's way and neither one makes it

the rest were treated with the amino acids, using 12 g 3 times a day for a 2-week period and then reducing the dose to 6 g 3 times a day. At 3 months, 56% of the treated participants had either reduced or completely eliminated symptoms of nocturia (versus 15% of the placebo group); 66% reported lessening of urgency (versus 11% on placebo, with 7% actually worsening); 43% had reduced frequency (15% of placebo group); and hesitancy was alleviated for half (as opposed to none of those on placebo).

Two further studies, both double-blind and placebo-controlled, were performed in the early 1970s in Japan and found similar results.[20,21] No side effects were seen in any of the studies. Unfortunately, this promising option appears inside. Then, instead of having two superheroes to fight for justice, you may have none at all. Similarly, two herbs for BPH may block each other from occupying receptor sites, producing a reduced instead of an enhanced effect.

Similarly, combining pharmaceutical medicines with herbs can also be counterproductive. No studies have been done on either the efficacy or the safety of such combinations. If taken together, the two treatments might interfere with each other's effectiveness or even produce unknown side effects. Remember that the naturally occurring chemicals in herbal preparations can act on receptors and enzymes just like synthetic pharmaceuticals; contrary to the belief of some, herbs, such as saw palmetto, are not magical but are surprisingly similar to drugs.

to have languished for over 20 years for reasons that are unclear. It clearly deserves further study.

As common ingredients in foods, these amino acids are not believed to be toxic. However, you should use the highest quality amino acid products when taking a supplement in high doses, because even very minor manufacturing contaminants may conceivably reach dangerous levels with these doses.

Essential Fatty Acids: Healthful, But Do They Help the Prostate?

Essential fatty acids (EFAs) are fatty acids that must be consumed regularly. Our bodies can't manufacture them, and we require them as building blocks for vital structures. They have been shown to play a role in maintaining immune system function, vision, and the formation of cell membranes.[22] Substances known as prostaglandins and leukotrienes are made from essential fatty acids found in the diet. Since these substances play a central role in inflammation, dietary supplementation with EFAs has been proposed as a treatment for many inflammatory conditions. These include rheumatoid arthritis, psoriasis, and multiple sclerosis.

You may recall from chapter 6 that inflammation appears to play a role in BPH as well. It may not be a coincidence that many of the plants used in the treatment of BPH contain large amounts of essential fatty acids, such as linoleic acid. Other good dietary sources of these acids are fatty fish (such as salmon and tuna) and canola and soybean oils. Pumpkin seeds are high not only in linoleic acid but also in zinc.

Unfortunately, there is little direct evidence that essential fatty acid supplementation can improve symptoms of BPH, except for one old and poorly performed study.[23] The only other "evidence" for the effectiveness of essential fatty acids for treatment of BPH is the fact that the lowest incidence of BPH worldwide occurs in Japan, where diets tend to be high in fish. This, of course, is not really conclusive evidence.

QUICK
REVIEW

- Saw palmetto is not the only natural treatment for BPH. Other herbal remedies with scientific evidence of positive effects on BPH symptoms include *Pygeum africanus* extract, nettle root extract, grass pollen extract, and the beta-sitosterol–containing portion of plant extracts (often from *Hypoxis rooperi*). For a discussion of safety issues with these treatments, see the chapter.

- The recommended dosage for pygeum is 100 to 200 mg daily.
- If using whole nettle root to make tea, use 4 to 6 g daily; if taking the extract, the recommended dosage is 600 to 1,200 mg daily.
- Grass pollen extract and beta-sitosterol are not yet widely available in the United States. The standard dosage of beta-sitosterol is 60 to 130 mg daily.
- Pumpkin seed as well as a number of dietary supplements, including zinc, a combination of amino acids (L-glutamic acid, L-alanine, and glycine), and essential fatty acids, have also been proposed as treatments of BPH symptoms, but the scientific evidence for the effectiveness of these treatments is weak to non-existent.
- The safety and efficacy of herb-herb and herb-drug combinations is not known. It is quite possible that separate treatments might counteract each other or cause undesirable side effects.

CHAPTER
ELEVEN

Putting It All Together

or your easy reference, this chapter contains a brief summary of key information contained in this book. Please refer to earlier chapters for more comprehensive information, including a detailed discussion of safety issues.

Benign Prostatic Hyperplasia

Saw palmetto is a well-accepted therapy for benign prostatic hyperplasia (BPH) in Europe. BPH is a noncancerous but excessive growth of the gland that lies just below the bladder, surrounding the urethra. The signs and symptoms of BPH include decreased force and stream of urine, postvoid dribbling, hesitancy, interrupted stream/intermittency, urinary retention, straining, increased urinary frequency, nocturia, dysuria, hematuria, urgency, and acute urinary retention. Although not life-threatening in the modern world, it can still become very uncomfortable, and certain symptoms can be serious if not treated.

If you're experiencing the symptoms described previously, you need to visit your doctor to get a diagnosis, because cancer of the prostate and BPH have identical symptoms. Prostate cancer is quite treatable if found early, but it can be fatal if left untreated. Unfortunately, saw palmetto is not an effective treatment for prostate cancer.

Conventional Treatments

Surgeries and procedures have been the main methods of treatment for BPH for at least the last 40 to 50 years. However, except in severe cases, drugs or herbal alternatives might be a preferable form of treatment.

The pharmaceutical drugs available for treatment of BPH are safe and effective, but they have drawbacks, too. Hytrin and Cardura are fast-acting but they can cause dizziness and fainting. Flomax is also fast-acting, but it can cause problems with ejaculation. Proscar is almost side-effect free, but it is slow-acting and may cause sexual dysfunction. Another problem with Proscar is that it can artificially lower PSA levels, which could mask the development of prostate cancer. Furthermore, Proscar only seems to work well in men with very big prostates (this does not necessarily mean those with the most severe BPH). On the plus side, Proscar is the only treatment that has been proven to reduce the need for surgery.

Saw Palmetto

Saw palmetto is a viable alternative to these medications. Controlled, double-blind, clinical studies involving a total of more than 1,700 participants have been performed to test its effectiveness. While there are still some holes in the research, the evidence strongly suggests that saw palmetto is an effective treatment for BPH and is approximately as effective as standard medications. Saw palmetto causes less severe side effects than Hytrin, Cardura, and Flomax, and it offers two big advantages over Proscar: It neither causes sexual dysfunction nor lowers PSA. However, unlike Proscar, we do not know if saw palmetto can reduce the need for surgery.

The recommended dosage of saw palmetto is 320 mg daily of an extract standardized to contain 85 to 95% fatty acids and sterols. You can take this as one daily dose or divide it into two parts. Taking more than the recommended dose will not give you additional benefits.

Saw palmetto appears to be quite safe. Its only documented side effect is mild stomach upset, which seems to be relieved in most cases by taking the extract with food. However, it's not recommended that you combine saw palmetto with standard drugs used for BPH, as they might counteract one another or cause undesirable side effects.

Other Natural Treatments for BPH

Saw palmetto is not the only natural treatment for BPH. Other herbal remedies with scientific evidence of positive effects on BPH symptoms include ***Pygeum africanus* extract, nettle root extract, grass pollen extract,** and the **beta-sitosterol–containing portion of plant extracts** (often from *Hypoxis rooperi*). For a discussion of safety issues with these treatments, see chapter 10.

The recommended dosage for pygeum is 100 to 200 mg daily. If you are using whole nettle root to make tea, use 4 to 6 g daily; if taking the extract, the recommended dosage is 600 to 1,200 mg daily. Grass pollen extract and beta-sitosterol are not yet widely available in the United States, but may provide effective relief.

Pumpkin seed as well as a number of dietary supplements, including zinc, a combination of amino acids (L-glutamic acid, L-alanine, and glycine), and essential fatty acids, have also been proposed as treatments of BPH symptoms, but the scientific evidence for the effectiveness of these treatments is weak to non-existent.

No matter which therapy you decide on, regular check-ups with your doctor will continue to be necessary to monitor your progress and to screen for prostate cancer.

Notes

Chapter One

1. Zomlefer WB. Guide to flowering plant families. Chapel Hill, NC: University of North Carolina Press, 1994: 306–308.

2. Wood HC and Osol A. The dispensatory of the United States of America, 23rd ed. Philadelphia: J. B. Lippincott Company, 1943: 971.

3. Hyam R and Pankhurst R. Plants and their names. New York: Oxford University Press, 1995: vii–viii, 425, 461.

4. Raven P, et al. Biology of plants, 4th ed. New York: Worth Publishers, Inc., 1986: 49–50, 63.

5. Tyler VE. Herbs of choice. Binghampton, NY: Worth Publishers, Inc., 1994: 82.

6. Wood HC and Osol A. 1943.

7. Krochmal A and Krochmal C. A guide to the medicinal plants of the United States. New York: Quadrangle/The New York Times Book Co., 1973: 204–205.

Chapter Two

1. Marieb EN. Human anatomy and physiology, 2nd ed. Redwood City, CA: The Benjamin/Cummings Publishing Company, Inc., 1992: 936.

2. Walsh P, et al. Campbell's urology, 7th ed. Philadelphia: W. B. Saunders Company, 1998: 110–113.

3. Briley M, et al. Inhibitory effect of Permixon® on testosterone 5-alpha-reductase activity of the rat ventral prostate. *Br J Pharmacol* 83: 401–410, 1984.

4. Délos S, et al. Testosterone metabolism in primary cultures of human prostate epithelial cells and fibroblasts. *J Steroid Biochem* 55(3/4): 375–383, 1995.

5. Iehlé C, et al. Human prostatic steroid 5-alpha-reductase isoforms—A comparative study of selective inhibitors. *J Steroid Biochem* 54(5/6): 273–279, 1995.

6. Ravenna L, et al. Effects of the lipidosterolic extract of *Serenoa repens* (Permixon®) on human prostatic cell lines. *Prostate* 29: 219–230, 1996.

7. Weisser H, et al. Effects of the *Sabal serrulata* extract IDS 89 and its subfractions on 5-alpha-reductase activity in human benign prostatic hyperplasia. *Prostate* 28: 300–306, 1996.

8. Kissane JM, ed. Anderson's pathology, 9th ed. St. Louis, MO: Mosby, 1990: 906.

9. Walsh P, et al. 1998.

10. American Cancer Society. Cancer facts and figures—1998. Atlanta, GA: American Cancer Society, 1998.

11. Carraro JC, et al. Comparison of phytotherapy (Permixon®) with finasteride in the treatment of benign prostate hyperplasia: A randomized international study of 1,098 patients. *Prostate* 29(4): 231–240, 1996.

12. Berkow R (ed.). The Merck manual, 15th ed. Rahway, NJ: Merck Sharp & Dohme Research Laboratories, 1987: 1564.

13. Hansen MV, et al. The agreement among urological experts on the diagnostic management of patients with common urological problems. *Br J Urol* 80(5): 787–792, 1997.

Chapter Three

1. Walsh P, et al. Campbell's urology, 7th ed. Philadelphia: W. B. Saunders Company, 1998: 1432–1442.

2. Briley M, et al. Inhibitory effect of Permixon® on testosterone 5-alpha-reductase activity of the rat ventral prostate. *Br J Pharmacol* 83: 401–410, 1984.

3. Délos S, et al. Testosterone metabolism in primary cultures of human prostate epithelial cells and fibroblasts. *J Steroid Biochem* 55(3/4): 375–383, 1995.

4. Iehlé C, et al. Human prostatic steroid 5-alpha-reductase isoforms—A comparative study of selective inhibitors. *J Steroid Biochem* 54(5/6): 273–279, 1995.

5. Ravenna L, et al. Effects of the lipidosterolic extract of *Serenoa repens* (Permixon®) on human prostatic cell lines. *Prostate* 29: 219–230, 1996.

6. Weisser H, et al. Effects of the *Sabal serrulata* extract IDS 89 and its subfractions on 5-alpha-reductase activity in human benign prostatic hyperplasia. *Prostate* 28: 300–306, 1996.

7. Walsh P, et al. 1998: 1435

8. Walsh P, et al. 1998: 1434

9. Carilla E, et al. Binding of Permixon, a new treatment for prostatic benign hyperplasia, to the cytosolic androgen receptor in the rat prostate. *J Steroid Biochem* 20(1): 521–523, 1984.

10. DiSilverio F, et al. Evidence that *Serenoa repens* extract displays an antiestrogenic activity in prostatic tissue of benign prostatic hypertrophy patients. *Eur Urol* 21: 309–314, 1992.

11. Walsh P, et al. 1998: 1435

12. Paubert-Braquet M, et al. Effect of the lipidic lipidosterolic extract of *Serenoa repens* (Permixon®) on the ionophore A23187-stimulated production of leukotriene B4 (LTB4) from human polymorphonuclear neutrophils. *Prostaglandins Leukotr Essent Fatty Acids* 57(3): 299–304, 1997.

13. Gutiérrez M, et al. Mechanisms involved in the spasmolytic effect of extracts from *Sabal serrulata* fruit on smooth muscle. *Gen Pharmacol* 27(1): 171–176, 1996.

14. Gutiérrez M, et al. Spasmolytic activity of a lipidic extract from *Sabal serrulata* fruits: Further study of the mechanisms underlying this activity. *Planta Med* 62: 507–511, 1996.

Chapter Four

1. Wershub LP. Urology: From antiquity to the 20th century. Saint Louis, MO: Warren H. Green, Inc., 1970.

2. Vogel VJ. American Indian medicine. Norman, Oklahoma: University of Oklahoma Press, 1970.

3. Shelley HS. The enlarged prostate: A brief history of its treatment. *J History Med Allied Sci* 24(4): 452–473, 1969.

4. Iverson HG and Foged P. The treatment of prostatic hyperplasia then and now in the Municipal Hospital Service of Copenhagen. *Acta Chir Scand* 433(Suppl.): 50–61, 1973.

5. Walsh P, et al. Campbell's urology, 7th ed. Philadelphia: W.B. Saunders Company, 1998: 1433–1442.

6. Walsh P, et al. 1998.

7. Mushinski M. Average charges for a radical prostatectomy and a transurethral resection of the prostate (TURP): Geographic variations, 1994. *Stat Bull Metrop Insur Co* 77(3): 19–27, 1996.

8. Walsh P, et al. 1998.

9. Walsh P, et al. 1998.

10. Hugosson J, et al. Outpatient transurethral incision of the prostate under local anesthesia: Operative results, patient security and cost effectiveness. *Scand J Urol Nephrol* 27(3): 381–385, 1993.

11. Cornford PA, et al. Daycase transurethral incision of the prostate using the holmium: YAG laser: Initial experience. *Br J Urol* 79(3): 383–384, 1997.

12. Riehmann M, et al. Transurethral resection versus incision of the prostate: A randomized, prospective study. *Urology* 45(5): 768–775, 1995.

13. Sparwasser C, et al. Long-term results of transurethral prostate incision (TUIP) and transurethral prostate resection (TURP). A prospective randomized study. *Urologe A* 34(2): 153–157, 1995.

14. Walsh P, et al. 1998.

15. Nawrocki JD, et al. A randomized controlled trial of transurethral microwave thermotherapy. *Br J Urol* 79(3): 389–393, 1997.

16. Rosario DJ, et al. Safety and efficacy of transurethral needle ablation of the prostate for symptomatic outlet obstruction. *Br J Urol* 80(4): 579–586, 1997.

17. Steele GS and Sleep DJ. Transurethral needle ablation of the prostate: A urodynamic-based study with 2-year followup. *J Urol* 158(5): 1834–1838, 1997.

18. Roehrborn CG, et al. Transurethral needle ablation for benign prostatic hyperplasia: 12-month results of a prospective multicenter U.S. study. *Urology* 51(3): 415–421, 1998.

Chapter Five

1. Wood HC and Osol A. The United States dispensatory. Philadelphia: J. B. Lippincott Company, 1943: 971–972.

2. Grayhack JT, et al. (eds.) Benign prostatic hyperplasia: NIAMDD Workshop Proceedings, February 20–21, 1975: 91.

3. Physicians' desk reference, 52nd ed. Montvale, NJ: Medical Economics Company, Inc., 1998: 449.

4. Walsh P, et al. Campbell's urology, 7th ed. Philadelphia: W. B. Saunders Company, 1998: 1460–1472.

5. Walsh P, et al. 1998.

6. Gormley GJ, et al. The effect of finasteride in men with benign prostatic hyperplasia. *N Engl J Med* 327: 1185–1191, 1992.

7. The Finasteride Study Group. Finasteride (MK-906) in the treatment of benign prostatic hyperplasia. *Prostate* 22: 291–299, 1993.

8. Lepor H, et al. The efficacy of terazosin, finasteride, or both in benign prostatic hyperplasia. *N Engl J Med* 335: 533–539, 1996.

9. Walsh PC. Editorial: Treatment of benign prostatic hyperplasia. *N Engl J Med* 335(8): 586–587, 1996.

10. McConnell JD, et al. The effect of finasteride on the risk of acute urinary retention and the need for surgical treatment among men with benign prostatic hyperplasia. Finasteride Long-Term Efficacy and Safety Study Group. *N Engl J Med.* 338(9): 557–563, 1998.

11. Guess HA, et al. The effect of finasteride on prostate specific antigen: Review of available data. *J Urol* 155: 3, 1996.

12. Pannek J, et al. Influence of finasteride on free and total serum prostate-specific antigen levels in men with benign prostatic hyperplasia. *J Urol* 159: 449–453, 1998.

13. Masters JG, et al. Free/total serum prostate-specific antigen ratio: How helpful is it in detecting prostate cancer? *Br J Urol* 81: 419–423, 1998.

14. Oesterling JE, et al. Biologic variability of prostate-specific antigen and its usefulness as a marker for prostate cancer: Effects of finasteride. The Finasteride PSA Study Group. *Urology* 50(1): 13–18, 1997.

15. Walsh P, et al. 1998.

16. McConnell JD, et al. 1998.

Chapter Six

1. Carraro JC, et al. Comparison of phytotherapy (Permixon®) with finasteride in the treatment of benign prostate hyperplasia: A randomized international study of 1,098 patients. *Prostate* 29: 231–240, 1996.

2. Plosker GL and Brogden RN. *Serenoa repens* (Permixon®): A review of its pharmacology and therapeutic effectiveness in benign prostatic hyperplasia. *Drugs Aging* 9(5): 379–395, 1996.

3. Champault G, et al. A double-blind trial of an extract of the plant *Serenoa repens* in benign prostatic hyperplasia. *Br J Clin Pharmacol* 18: 461–462, 1984.

4. Plosker GL and Brogden RN. 1996.

5. Descotes JL, et al. Placebo-controlled evaluation of the efficacy and tolerability of Permixon® in benign prostatic hyperplasia after exclusion of placebo responders. *Clin Drug Invest* 9: 291–297, 1995.

6. Reece Smith H, et al. The value of Permixon in benign prostatic hypertrophy. *Br J Urol* 58: 36–40, 1986.

7. Nickel JC. Placebo therapy of benign prostatic hyperplasia: A 25-month study. *Br J Urol* 81: 383–387, 1998.

8. Carraro JC, et al. 1996.

9. Braeckman J. The extract of *Serenoa repens* in the treatment of benign prostatic hyperplasia: A multicenter open study. *Curr Ther Res* 55(7): 776–785, 1994.

10. Romics I, et al. Experience in treating benign prostatic hypertrophy with *Sabal serrulata* for one year. *Int Urol Nephrol* 25: 565–569, 1993.

11. Sultan C, et al. Inhibition of androgen metabolism and binding by a liposterolic extract of "*Serenoa repens* B" in human foreskin fibroblasts. *J Steroid Biochem* 20(1): 515–519, 1984.

12. Carilla E, et al. Binding of Permixon, a new treatment for prostatic benign hyperplasia, to the cytosolic androgen receptor in the rat prostate. *J Steroid Biochem* 20(1): 521–523, 1984.

13. Iehlé C, et al. Human prostatic steroid 5-alpha-reductase isoforms—a comparative study of selective inhibitors. *J Steroid Biochem Mol Biol* 54(5/6): 273–279, 1995.

14. Délos S, et al. Testosterone metabolism in primary cultures of human prostate epithelial cells and fibroblasts. *J Steroid Biochem Mol Biol* 55(3/4): 375–383, 1995.

15. Niederprüm H-J, Schweikert H-U, Zänker KS. Testosterone 5-alpha-reductase inhibition by free fatty acids from *Sabal serrulata* fruits. *Phytomedicine* 1: 127–133, 1994.

16. Strauch G, et al. Comparison of finasteride (Proscar®) and *Serenoa repens* (Permixon®) in the inhibition of 5-alpha-reductase in healthy male volunteers. *Eur Urol* 26(3): 247–252, 1994.

17. Plosker GL and Brogden RN. 1996.

18. Bombardelli E and Morazzoni P. *Serenoa repens*. As cited in *Fitoterapia* 68(2): 99–113, 1997.

19. Ravenna L, et al. Effects of the lipidosterolic extract of *Serenoa repens* (Permixon®) on human prostatic cell lines. *Prostate* 29: 219–230, 1996.

20. DiSilverio F, et al. Evidence that *Serenoa repens* extract displays an antiestrogenic activity in prostatic tissue of benign prostatic hypertrophy patients. *Eur Urol* 21: 309–314, 1992.

21. DiSilvero F, et al. 1992.

22. Gutiérrez M, et al. Mechanisms involved in the spasmolytic effect of extracts from *Sabal serrulata* fruit on smooth muscle. *Gen Pharmacol* 27(1): 171–176, 1996.

23. Gutiérrez M, et al. Spasmolytic activity of a lipidic extract from *Sabal serrulata* fruits: Further study of the mechanisms underlying this activity. *Planta Med* 62: 507–511, 1996.

24. Paubert-Braquet M, et al. Effect of the lipidic lipidosterolic extract of *Serenoa repens* (Permixon®) on the ionophore A23187-stimulated production of leukotriene B4 (LTB4) from human polymorphonuclear neutrophils. *Prostaglandins Leukot Essent Fatty Acids* 57(3): 299–304, 1997.

25. Paubert-Braquet M, et al. 1997.

26. Powers JE. That pesky prostate and the saw palmetto. *SDJ Med* 50: 453–454, 1997.

Chapter Seven

1. Braeckman J, et al. Efficacy and safety of the extract of *Serenoa repens* in the treatment of benign prostatic hyperplasia: The therapeutic equivalence between twice and once daily dosage forms. *Phytother Res* 11(8): 558–563, 1997.

2. Plosker GL and Brogden, RN. *Serenoa repens* (Permixon®): A review of its pharmacology and therapeutic efficacy in benign prostatic hyperplasia. *Drugs & Aging* 9(5): 379–395, 1996.

3. Cristoni A, et al. Chemical and pharmacological study on hypercritical CO_2 extracts of *Serenoa repens* fruits. *Fitoterapia* 68(4): 355–358, 1997.

4. Bach D, Schmitt M, and Ebeling L. Phytopharmaceutical and synthetic agents in the treatment of benign prostatic hyperplasia (BPH). *Phytomedicine* 3(4): 309–313, 1996/97.

5. Carraro JC, et al. Comparison of phytotherapy (Permixon®) with finasteride in the treatment of benign prostate hyperplasia: A randomized international study of 1,098 patients. *Prostate* 29: 231–240, 1996.

Chapter Eight

1. Plosker GL and Brogden RN. *Serenoa repens* (Permixon®): A review of its pharmacology and therapeutic efficacy in benign prostatic hyperplasia. *Drugs & Aging* 9(5): 379–395, 1996.

2. Plosker GL and Brogden RN. 1996.

3. Bach D, Schmitt M, and Ebeling L. Phytopharmaceutical and synthetic agents in the treatment of benign prostatic hyperplasia (BPH). *Phytomedicine* 3(4): 309–313, 1996–1997.

4. Romics I, et al. Experience in treating benign prostatic hypertrophy with *Sabal serrulata* for one year. *Int Urol Nephrol* 25(6): 565–569, 1993.

5. Carraro JC, et al. Comparison of phytotherapy (Permixon®) with finasteride in the treatment of benign prostate hyperplasia: A randomized international study of 1,098 patients. *Prostate* 29: 231–240, 1996.

6. Bombardelli E and Morazzoni P. *Serenoa repens*. As cited in *Fitoterapia* 68(2): 99–113, 1997.

7. Plosker GL and Brogden RN. 1996.

8. Schulz, V, et al. Rational phytotherapy. New York: Springer-Verlag, 1998: 228.

9. Blumenthal M. The complete Commission E monographs. Boston: American Botanical Council, 1998: 201.

10. Walsh P, et al. Campbell's urology, 7th ed. Philadelphia: W. B. Saunders Company, 1998: 1443.

11. Braeckman J. The extract of *Serenoa repens* in the treatment of benign prostatic hyperplasia: A multicenter open study. *Curr Ther Res* 55(7): 776–785, 1994.

12. Carraro JC, et al. 1996.

13. Trabucco, AF. Saw palmetto warning: Problems with detecting prostate cancer. *Oncology Times: The Independent Newspaper for Cancer Specialists.* 19(1): 5–6, Jan. 1997.

Chapter Nine

1. Carraro JC, et al. Comparison of phytotherapy (Permixon®) with finasteride in the treatment of benign prostate hyperplasia: A randomized international study of 1,098 patients. *Prostate* 29(4): 231–240, 1996.

2. Physicians' desk reference, 52nd ed. Montvale, NJ: Medical Economics Company, Inc., 1998: 719.

3. Carraro JC, et al. 1996.

4. Shulz V, et al. Rational phytotherapy. New York: Springer-Verlag, 1998: 233.

Chapter Ten

1. Bombardelli E and Morazonni P. *Prunus africanus.* *Fitoterapia* 68(3): 205–218, 1997.

2. Schulz V, et al. Rational phytotherapy. New York: Springer-Verlag, 1998: 233.

3. Hobbs C. Foundations of health. Capitola, CA: Botanica Press, 1992: 49.

4. ESCOP monographs. Fascicule 3 *Urticae radix*. Exeter, UK: 1997.

5. Hartmann RW, Mark M, and Soldati F. Inhibition of 5-alpha-reductase and aromatase by PHL-00801 (Prostonin®), a combination of PY 102 (*Pygeum africanum*) and UR 102 (*Urtica dioica*) extracts. *Phytomedicine* 3(2): 121–128, 1996.

6. Krzeski T, et al. Combined extracts of *Urtica dioica* and *Pygeum africanus* in the treatment of benign prostatic hyperplasia: Double-blind comparison of two doses. *Clin Ther* 15(6): 1011–1020, 1993.

7. Schulz V, et al. 1998: 228–229.

8. ESCOP monographs. 1997.

9. Buck AC, et al. Treatment of outflow tract obstruction due to benign prostatic hyperplasia with the pollen extract, Cernilton. A double-blind, placebo-controlled study. *Br J Urol* 66(4): 398–404, 1990.

10. Schulz, V, et al. 1998: 229–230.

11. Maekawa M, et al. Clinical evaluation of Cernilton on benign prostatic hypertrophy—a multiple center double-blind study with Paraprost. *Hinyokika Kiyo* 36(4): 495–516, 1990.

12. Dutkiewicz S. Usefulness of Cernilton in the treatment of benign prostatic hyperplasia. *Int Urol Nephrol* 28(1): 49–53, 1996.

13. Schulz V, et al. 1998.

14. Berges RR, et al. Randomised, placebo-controlled double-blind clinical trial of beta-sitosterol in patients with benign prostatic hyperplasia. Beta-sitosterol Study Group. *Lancet* 345(8964): 1529–1532, 1995.

15. Schulz V, et al. 1998: 231–232.

16. Schulz V, et al. 1998: 229–230.

17. Blumenthal M. The complete Commission E monographs. Boston: American Botanical Council, 1998: 193.

18. Berman E, et al. Zinc: A key urological element. Poster presentation, American Urological Association annual meeting, Chicago, 1974.

19. Dumrau F. Benign prostatic hyperplasia: Amino acid therapy for symptomatic relief. *Am J Geriatr* 10: 426–430, 1962.

20. Shimaya M and Sugiura H. Double-blind test of PPC for prostatic hyperplasia. *Hinyokika Kiyo* 16(5): 231–236, 1970.

21. Aito K and Iwatsubo E. The conservative treatment of prostatic hypertrophy with Paraprost. *Hinyokika Kiyo* 18(1): 41–44, 1972.

22. Wardlaw GM and Insel PM. Perspectives in nutrition, 2nd ed. St. Louis, MO: Mosby-Year Book, Inc., 1993: 104–105.

23. Hart JP and Cooper WL. Vitamin F in the treatment of prostatic hyperplasia. Report No. 1, Milwaukee, WI: Lee Foundation for Nutritional Research, 1941.

Index

A

Abnormal ejaculation, *see* Retrograde ejaculation
Adrenaline, 71
Adrenergic hormones, 71
Aging, 18, 37
Alcohol
  consumption, 23
  use in extraction, *see* Extracts, ethyl alcohol
Alpha-1 blockers, *see* Alpha-adrenergic blockers
Alpha-1A blockers, *see* Alpha-adrenergic blockers
Alpha-1 receptors, *see* Alpha-adrenergic receptors
Alpha-adrenergic blockers
  compared to saw palmetto, 125–127, 129
  types of, 46–47, 70–76
Alpha-adrenergic receptors, 46–47, 71–76
American dwarf palm, *see* Saw palmetto
American Urological Association Symptom Index, 52

Amino acids, 145–147
Androgen hormones, 17, 40, 42, 97
Androgen receptors, 17, 40, 42
Anesthesia
  and surgical procedures, 57
  and urinary retention, 23
Antiandrogenics, 70
Anticholinergics, 23
Antihistamines, 23
Apoptosis, *see* Cells, death, programmed
AR, *see* Androgen receptors
Arecaceae family, 3
Assessment questionnaires, 52–53
Asthenia, 73–74
AUA, *see* American Urological Association Symptom Index

B

Bed-wetting, *see* Enuresis
Benadryl, 23
Benign prostatic hyperplasia
  asymptomatic, 24–25
  causes of, 37–48

Benign prostatic hyperplasia (*continued*)
 death resulting from, 25
 degree of enlargement, 24–25
 diagnosis of, 26–35
 prevalence, 11
 smooth muscle involvement, 46–47, 97–98
 symptoms of, 18–25
  measuring, 52–53, 86
 treatment
  catheterization, 49–50, 66
  drugs, 69–83, 125–133
  herbs, 6–8, 85–144
  history of, 49–52
  laser therapy, 58, 62–63
  surgical, 49–68
  watchful waiting, 56
Benign prostatic hypertrophy, 39
Beta-adrenergic hormone receptors, 71–72
Beta-sitosterol, 138, 142–143
Biopsy, 33–34
Bladder
 cancer, 22
 emptying of, 20
 infection, 7, 22, 27
 trabeculation, 21
Bladder neck contracture, 57
Bleeding, 56, 58
Blood clots, 58
Blood in urine, *see* Hematuria
Boyarsky's symptom score, 52
BPH, *see* Benign prostatic hyperplasia
Bratman, Steve, 80–81, 100–102

Breast enlargement, 80
British Journal of Clinical Pharmacology, 91
British Journal of Urology, 34, 79, 93

C

Campbell's Urology, 19, 60, 75
Cancer
 bladder, 22
 prostate, *see* Prostate, cancer
Cannula, 50
Capsule, *see* Prostate
Cardura
 compared to saw palmetto, 125–127
 cost, 82, 131–132
 role in treating BPH, 47, 70–74
 side effects, 73–74, 129
Castration, 37–38, 69–70
Catheterization
 balloon, 66
 historical use of, 49–50
 and surgical procedures, 56
Cells
 communication among, 43
 creation of, 40–41, 43–45
 in culture, 44–45
 death, programmed, 40–41
 hyperplastic prostate, 42
 inflammatory, 43–45, 98–99
 mitosis, 41
Central zone, *see* Prostate, zones
Cholesterol, 6
Coagulation necrosis, 62–63

Commission E Monograph, 119, 140, 144
Computerized tomography, 33
Corn pollen, *see* Grass pollen
Creatinine, 30
CT, *see* Computerized tomography
Cystitis, 61
Cystogram, 33
Cystoscope, 51–52
Cystoscopy, 32

D

Death
  from BPH, 25
  of prostate cells, 40–41
Decongestants, 23
DHT, *see* Dihydrotestosterone
Difficulty breathing, *see* Dyspnea
Digital rectal exam, 27–29
Digoxin, 62
Dihydrotestosterone
  and Proscar, 76
  and pumpkin seed, 143–144
  role in prostate growth, 17, 38–42
  and saw palmetto, 40, 95–97
Diphenhydramine, *see* Benadryl
Dispensatory of the United States of America, The, 7, 69
Dizziness, 73
DNA,
  in apoptosis, 41
  and dihydrotestosterone, 40

Doxazosin, *see* Cardura
DRE, *see* Digital rectal exam
Dribbling, 19
Drowsiness, 74
Drugs, *see* specific drugs
Drugs & Aging, 90
Dynamic obstruction, 46
Dyspnea, 74
Dysuria, 22

E

Edema, 74
EFA, *see* Essential fatty acids
Egyptians, 49–50
Ejaculatory disorder, 80
Ejaculatory ducts, 16
Electrovaporization, 63–64
Embryonic reawakening, 43
Enlargement of prostate, *see* Benign prostatic hyperplasia
Enuresis, 22
Epididymitis, 61, 65
Epinephrine, 71
ESCOP, *see* European Scientific Cooperative on Phytotherapy
Essential fatty acids, 147–148
Estrogen, 42, 97
Ethyl alcohol, 108
European Scientific Cooperative on Phytotherapy, 140
Experimental design, 44–45
Extracts
  ethyl alcohol, 108
  hexane, 108
  liquefied CO_2, 108–109

Extracts (*continued*)
   methods of production,
      105–106, 108–109
Extravasation, 55

F

Fatigue, 73
Fatty acids
   description, 5
   essential, 147–148
   interaction with
      testosterone, 95–96
Ferguson, William, 50–51
Fiber optics, 52
Finasteride, *see* Proscar
5-alpha-reductase, 17,
      39–40, 95
Flomax
   compared to saw palmetto,
      125–127
   cost, 82, 131–132
   role in treating BPH, 47, 70,
      74–75
   side effects, 75, 129
Fluid retention, *see* edema
Force of urinary stream, 19

G

Germany
   Commission E Monograph,
      119
   use of herbal remedies
      beta-sitosterol, 142
      frequency, 8
      grass pollen, 140–141
      nettle root, 140
      saw palmetto, 85
GF, *see* Growth factors

Glandular tissue, 16, 46–47
Glycine, 145
Grass pollen
   and prostate cancer, 141
   role in treating BPH, 140–141
   safety issues, 141–142
Growth factors, 43–45, 98–99

H

Headache, 74
Heart attack, 58
Hematuria, 22
Herbs, *see* specific herbs
Hesitancy, 19–20
Hexane, 108
High-intensity focused
      ultrasound, 65
History of North Carolina, 4
Hyperplasia, 39
Hyperthermia, 64–65
Hypertrophy, 39
Hypoechoic tissue, 31
Hypotension, 73–74
Hypoxis rooperi, see Beta-
      sitosterol
Hytrin
   compared to saw palmetto,
      125–127
   cost, 82, 131–132
   role in treating BPH, 47,
      70–74
   side effects, 73–74, 129

I

Impotence
   alpha-adrenergic blockers,
      74–75
   Proscar, 80–81

prostatectomy, 60
transurethral resection, 56
In vitro experiments, 44–45
In vivo experiments, 44–45
Incontinence
prostatectomy, 61
transurethral resection, 56
Indians, *see* Native Americans
Infertility, 55
Intermittency, *see*
Interrupted stream
International Prostate
Symptom Score, 52
Internet, 120, 121
Interrupted stream, 20
Intraurethral stents, 66
Intravenous pyelogram, 32–33
Iodine, 32
IPSS, *see* International
Prostate Symptom Score
IVP, *see* Intravenous pyelogram

J
Japan, 146, 148

K
Kidney failure, *see* Renal
insufficiency

L
L-alanine, 145
L-glutamic acid, 145
Laser therapy, 58, 62–63
Leukotrienes, 148
Libido, decreased, 80–81
Linoleic acid, 148
Low blood pressure, *see*
Hypotension

M
Magnetic resonance imaging, 33
Materia Medica Americana, 5
Mayans, 6
Mead, Susan, 100–101
Medicinal herbs, *see*
specific herbs
Medline, 120
Microwaves, 64
Mitosis, 41
MRI, *see* Magnetic resonance
imaging
Muscles
contractions, 46–47
detrusor, 20
relaxation, 97–98
smooth, 46, 97–98
urethral sphincter, 14, 19

N
Nasal congestion, 74
National Formulary, 6–7
Native Americans
use of catheterization, 49
use of medicinal herbs, 4–6
Nausea, 74
Nettle root
dosage, 140
role in treating BPH,
138–139
safety issues, 140
*New England Journal of
Medicine,* 78
Nighttime urination, *see*
Nocturia
Nocturia, 21
Nodularity, 28
Nonessential amino acids, 145

Nutritional supplements, *see* specific supplements

O

Oesterling, J.E., 60
Open prostatectomy, *see* prostatectomy
Orgasm, 13, 14, 55

P

Pain with urination, *see* Dysuria
Palmae family, 3
Paré, Ambroise, 50
PDR, see Physicians' Desk Reference
Peak flow rate, 53
Peripheral zone, *see* Prostate, zones
PFR, *see* Peak flow rate
Pharmaceutical drugs, *see* specific drugs
Pharmacopeia of the United States, The, 6
Phenylpropanolamine, 23
Physician's Desk Reference, 73, 119
Placebo effect, 93
Pollen, grass
  role in treating BPH, 140–141
  safety issues, 141–142
Postvoid dribbling, 19
Postvoid residual volume, 53
Poultices, 7
Powers, James E., 99
Progesterone, 97

Proliferation, *see* Cells, creation of
Proscar
  cancer detection, 78–80
  compared to saw palmetto, 125–129
  cost, 82, 131–132
  description, 70, 76–77
  dihydrotestosterone, 39–40, 75, 96
  effectiveness, 77–78
  prostate-specific antigen levels, 30, 78–80, 89, 131
  prostate volume, 77–78, 89–90, 128
  side effects, 80–81, 129–131
Prostaglandins, 148
Prostaglandins, Leukotrienes, and Essential Fatty Acids, 45
Prostate
  anatomy of, 12–16
  apex, 14
  base, 14
  boggy texture, 28
  cancer
    biopsies, 33–34
    detection, 79
    diagnosis, 35
    prostate-specific antigen levels, 29–30
    and saw palmetto, 35, 122–123
    self-treatment, 35
    survival rate, 25
    symptoms, 24

capsule, 16, 55–56
enlargement, *see* Benign
    prostatic hyperplasia
lobes, 14
location, 12
nodularity, 28
normal growth and
    development, 17–18,
    38–42
prostatitis, 28–29
size, 12
tissue types, 16
zones, 14–15
Prostate-specific antigens
bound, 30
complexed, 30
density, 29
free, 30
and Proscar, 78–80, 89
and saw palmetto, 89,
    120–121, 122–123
testing, 29–30
velocity, 29–30
Prostatectomy, 53, 58–62
Prostatic fluid
description, 16
in diagnosis of prostate
    infection, 28–29
function, 16
production, 43
Prostatism, 30
Prostatitis, 28–29
PSA, *see* Prostate-specific
    antigens
Pseudoephedrine, *see*
    Sudafed
Pumpkin seed, 143–144

PVR volume, *see* Postvoid
    residual volume
Pygeum africanus
dosage, 137–138
role in treating benign
    prostatic hyperplasia,
    136–138
role in treating prostate
    infection, 29
safety issues, 138

Q
Questionnaires, assessment,
    52–53

R
Radio-frequency waves, 64
Rational Phytotherapy, 140
Renal failure, *see* Renal
    insufficiency
Renal insufficiency, 24, 30, 32
Resectoscope, 51–52
Retrograde ejaculation
Flomax, 75
laser therapy, 63
prostatectomy, 60
transurethral resection, 54–55
Rye pollen, *see* Grass pollen

S
Sabal serrulata, see Saw
    palmetto
Saw palmetto
active ingredients, 105
anecdotal reports,
    110–114, 130
as antispasmodic, 47, 97–98

Saw palmetto (*continued*)
  compared with conventional
      medications, 125–133
  composition, 5–6
  cost, 82, 107, 131–132
  current use, 8, 85, 132
  description, 1–2
  dosage, 106–107
  drug interactions, 119
  effects
    dihydrotestosterone levels,
        40, 95–97
    inflammatory cells, 98–99
    prostate-specific antigen
        levels, 89, 120–123
    reduction of prostate size,
        89–90, 94–95
    sexual function, 89, 111–112
    smooth muscle, 97–98
  habitat, 1
  history of medical uses, 4–5,
      6–7
  mechanisms of action, 95–99
  nomenclature, 2–4
  open studies, 94–95
  placebo-controlled studies,
      90–93
  and prostate cancer, 35, 110,
      122–123
  safety issues, 117–123
  side effects, 117–118,
      129–131
  toxicity, 118–119
  uses, 6–8
  when not to take, 109–110
Schopf, Johann David, 5
Scrub palm, *see* Saw palmetto

Seminal fluids, 13
Seminal vesicles, 16
Serenoa repens, see Saw
    palmetto
Sex hormone–binding
    globulin (SHBG), 139
SHBG, *see* Sex hormone–
    binding globulin
Smith, Reece, 92
Solvents, 108–109
*South Dakota Journal of
    Medicine,* 99
Sperm, 13, 16, 61
Stents, 66
Sterol, 5–6
Stomach pains, 7
Straining, to pass urine, 21
Strangury, 22
Stroke, 58
Subacute cystitis, 7
Sudafed, 23
Surgery, *see* specific surgery
Supplements, *see* specific
    supplements
Sympathomimetic
    decongestants, 23

T
Tamoxifen, 97
Tamsulosin, *see* Flomax
Terazosin, *see* Hytrin
Testes
  and benign prostatic
      hyperplasia, 37–38, 70
  castration, 37–38
  epididymitis, 61
Testosterone, 17, 39–40, 42

Thermosensitive stents, 66
Thermotherapy, 64–65
Timothy pollen, *see* Grass pollen
Tissue, *see* specific tissues
Trabeculation, 21
Transcription, 40
Transition zone, *see* Prostate, zones
Transurethral incision of prostate, 53, 56–58
Transurethral needle ablation, 65–66
Transurethral resection of prostate, 52–56
Transurethral resection syndrome, 55
Tree of Life, The, 100
TRUS, *see* Ultrasound, transrectal
TUIP, *see* Transurethral incision of prostate
TUNA, *see* Transurethral needle ablation
Tunneling tools, 50
TURP, *see* Transurethral resection of prostate

U

Ultrasound
high-intensity focused, 65
transabdominal, 31–32
transducer, 31
transrectal, 31
United States Dispensatory, see Dispensatory of the United States of America, The

Urethra
description, 13
dynamic obstruction of, 46
narrowing of, 20–21
obstruction, 20–21, 46
sphincter, 14, 19
Urge incontinence, 22
Urgency, 22
Urinalysis, 27
Urinary frequency, 21
Urinary retention, 20
acute, 23–24
with hyperthermia and thermotherapy, 65
Urinary tract infection, 65
Urodynamics, 27

V

Van Wassenaer, Nicolaes, 4
Vaporization, 63
Vascularization, 22
Vas deferens, 16
Video imaging, 52
Voiding, 19

W

Watchful waiting, 25, 56

Z

Zinc
as nutritional supplement, 144–145
in prostatic fluid, 16
Zones, of the prostate, *see* Prostate

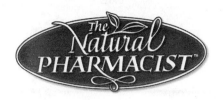

About the Author

Anna M. Barton holds a degree in biological sciences. Her background includes work in biomedical research laboratories, freelance writing, and medical transcription. Her familiarity with these areas, combined with painstaking research, allows her to provide reliable information about alternatives and adjuncts to the standard western medical approach.

About the Series Editors

Steven Bratman, M.D., medical director of Prima Health, has many years of experience in the alternative medicine field. A graduate of the University of California at Davis, Medical School, he has also trained in herbology, nutrition, Chinese medicine, and other alternative therapies, and has worked closely with a wide variety of alternative practitioners. He is the author of *The Natural Pharmacist: Your Complete Guide to Herbs* (Prima), *The Natural Pharmacist: Your Complete Guide to Illnesses and Their Natural Remedies* (Prima), *The Natural Pharmacist Guide to St. John's Wort and Depression* (Prima), *The Alternative Medicine Ratings Guide* (Prima), and *The Alternative Medicine Sourcebook* (Lowell House).

David J. Kroll, Ph.D., is a professor of pharmacology and toxicology at the University of Colorado School of Pharmacy and a consultant for pharmacists, physicians, and alternative practitioners on the indications and cautions for herbal medicine use. A graduate of both the University of Florida and the Philadelphia College of Pharmacy and Science, Dr. Kroll has lectured widely and has published articles in a number of medical journals, abstracts, and newsletters.

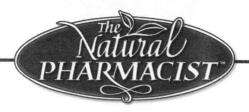

Inside—Find the Answers to These Questions and More

☑ How can saw palmetto help my prostate? (See page 87.)

☑ How much saw palmetto should I take? (See page 106.)

☑ How does saw palmetto compare to prescription drugs? (See page 125.)

☑ Does saw palmetto cause any side effects? (See page 117.)

☑ How long do I have to take it before I start seeing results? (See page 110.)

☑ Will taking saw palmetto affect my sex life? (See page 111.)

☑ What precautions should I take before using saw palmetto? (See page 35.)

☑ Can saw palmetto help reduce trips to the bathroom? (See page 90.)

☑ How can nettle, pygeum, beta-sitosterol, and other natural treatments help my prostate? (See page 135.)

THE NATURAL PHARMACIST Library

Arthritis

Diabetes

Echinacea and Immunity

Feverfew and Migraines

Garlic and Cholesterol

Ginkgo and Memory

Heart Disease Prevention

Herbs

Illnesses and Their Natural Remedies

Kava and Anxiety

Menopause

PMS

Reducing Cancer Risk

Saw Palmetto and the Prostate

St. John's Wort and Depression

Vitamins and Supplements

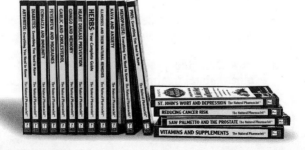